radiant
beauty

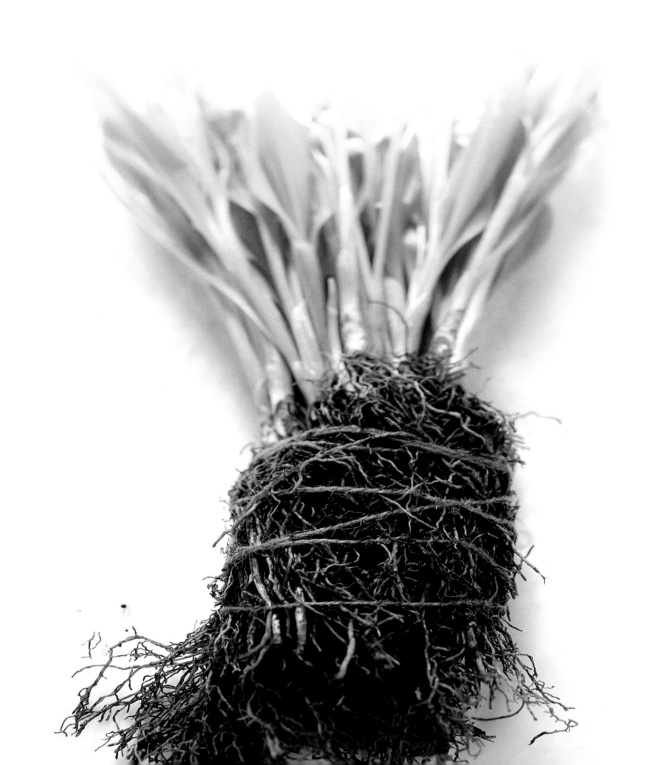

radiant *beauty*

Your Healthy and Organic Guide to Total Body Well-Being

MARY BETH JANSSEN

RODALE

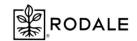

RODALE

WE **INSPIRE** AND **ENABLE** PEOPLE TO IMPROVE
THEIR LIVES AND THE WORLD AROUND THEM

We're always happy to hear from you. For questions or comments concerning the editorial content of this book, please write to:

Rodale Book Readers' Service
33 East Minor Street
Emmaus, PA 18098

Look for other Rodale books wherever books are sold. Or call us at (800) 848-4735.

For more information about Rodale Organic Living magazines and books, visit us at
www.organicstyle.com

Editor: Donna Shryer
Project Manager: Christine Bucks
Cover and Interior Book Designer: Christin Gangi
Contributing Designer: Dale Mack
Cover Photographer: Tara Sgroi
Cover Hair and Makeup: Sara Johnson with Sarah Laird, artist representative
Interior Illustrator: Martina Witte
Interior Photographer: Sang An
Interior Photo Stylist: Bobbi Lin
Photography Editor: Lyn Horst
Photography Assistant: Jackie L. Ney
Layout Designer: Jennifer H. Giandomenico
Researchers: Jennifer L. Bright and Diana Erney
Copy Editor: Erana Bumbardatore
Product Specialist: Jodi Schaffer
Indexer: Nanette Bendyna
Editorial Assistance: Kerrie A. Cadden and Susan L. Nickol

Rodale Organic Living Books

Editorial Director: Christopher Hirsheimer
Executive Creative Director: Christin Gangi
Executive Editor: Kathleen DeVanna Fish
Art Director: Patricia Field
Content Assembly Manager: Robert V. Anderson Jr.
Studio Manager: Leslie M. Keefe
Copy Manager: Nancy N. Bailey
Projects Coordinator: Kerrie A. Cadden

Library of Congress Cataloging-in-Publication Data

Janssen, Mary Beth.
    Radiant beauty : your healthy and organic guide to total body well-being / Mary Beth Janssen.
        p.   cm.
    Includes bibliographical references and index.
    ISBN 0–87596–926–7 (paperback)
    1. Beauty, Personal.   2. Herbal cosmetics.
3. Naturopathy.   4. Natural foods. I. Title.
RA776.98 .J36   2001
646.7—dc21   2001003703

Distributed in the book trade by St. Martin's Press

2   4   6   8   10   9   7   5   3   1   paperback

Health, Harmony, Organic Style!

Aren't the best moments in your life the ones when you feel most connected to the best in yourself, in harmony with nature, and with the world around you? When you do the right thing for others, yourself, and nature, you can't help but feel happy, satisfied, and at peace.

The choices you make can make your life more joyful. You can choose how to live, eat, travel, raise your family, work, and get in touch with your soul in ways that lead you to a better future and more moments of happiness . . . the moments that really matter the most.

The best choices for you are often the best choices for nature. Choices that preserve all that you love and need. Choices that help you lead a healthier life. Choices that leave you with a clean conscience and a happy heart.

The great news is that these days, the right choices can be beautiful, delicious, stylish, fun, and deeply satisfying. Let *Organic Style* magazine and books be your guide to doing the right thing and loving every minute of it.

Rodale has brought you the most important and inspiring information on healthy active organic living since 1942. Join us as *Organic Style* continues in this rich tradition.

Welcome to a future you *want* to live in!

Maria Rodale

Maria Rodale
Rodale Organic Style Books

To my beloved husband, James. As we travel through this life together, you continually inspire me with your devotion to all things organic. To my wonderful family, especially my parents, Nelly and Hubert. Your love and wisdom is a shining beacon in so many lives.

Contents

Acknowledgments

Thanks to Donna Shryer for her inspired editorial guidance, and to Fern Bradley, Christine Bucks, Chris Gangi, and the team at Rodale, for giving this book a beautiful look and feel.

Special thanks to all those who have been and continue to be an integral part of my spiritual unfolding: Dr. Deepak Chopra, Dr. David Simon, and all my dear friends at The Chopra Center for Well-Being; also Dr. Andrew Weil, Dr. Christiane Northrup, Dr. Candace Pert, Dr. Richard Gerber, Matthew Fox, Buster Yellow Kidney, Michael Harner, Ph.D., Fritof Capra, Thomas Berry, Rupert Sheldrake, Duane Elgin, and my dear friends at Compassion in Action and Women's Spirit Drummers.

Also thanks to those who have been mentors and advocates within the realm of holistic living, organicism, and beauty and wellness integration: Maria Rodale and the entire Rodale organization, Ronnie Cummins and the Organic Consumers Association, Christie Phillips, Jim Slama at Sustain, Althea Northage Orr and Patricia Howell, Don Spencer, David Raccuglia, Horst Rechelbacher, Aubrey Hampton, Linda Burmeister, Rachelle Geller, the Organic Trade Association, United Plant Savers, the Union of Concerned Scientists, the Integral Yoga Community, the Sivananda Yoga Vedanta Community, the Himalayan Institute, Wendell Berry, Rudoph Steiner, and Kenny Ausubel and the Bioneers.

Thanks to Faith Popcorn; you keep me clicking.

Special thanks to my physicians, Dr. Renee McMurry and Dr. Joseph Mercola.

Thanks to those who are my lifeblood within the beauty cosmos—Leo Passage, Vi Nelson, Gordon Miller, Greg and Joanne Starkman, my friends at MOP, Pivot Point International, the National Cosmetology Association, the American Beauty Association, The Salon Association, and behindthechair.com. Thanks to Mary Atherton and Michele Musgrove at *Modern Salon* magazine and to Robbin McClain at *American Salon* magazine.

Thanks to my friends and confidantes, Vi, Bea, Susan, Leslie, Lynn and Ellen. Susan, I truly appreciate your reading and commenting on this manuscript.

And, finally, thanks to all those who are striving to live a more simple, natural, and organic lifestyle—one that is in tune with nature, and thus spirit.

Finding Your Radiant Beauty

As Rodin so elegantly stated, "Beauty is but the spirit breaking through the flesh." I hope you discover the essence of this thought as you read this book. To help you find this point of enlightenment, I'd like to share some of my experiences with you—some of which happened in the past few years and others that occurred long ago, when I was a child. Together they represent a culmination of many years traveled along the path of radiant beauty and wellness.

Those I've met along the way know how strongly I believe in that old Latin aphorism, "By learning you will teach, by teaching you will learn." As a licensed educator for more than 25 years, I've had the richest of opportunities to teach as well as learn from many different people and their native cultures. I've found true enlightenment and inspiration in terraced rice paddies and temples of Indonesia, the Swiss Alps, English palaces and gardens, Germany's Black Forest, the ports of Hong Kong, many of Italy's beautiful cities, and Japan during apple blossom season.

As I enjoyed many of these adventures back in the 1980s, I recognized a shift taking place in the beauty profession—a change that I now know was the precursor to today's enlightened spa culture. What I was witnessing was a welcome (and healthy!) blurring of the lines that had traditionally separated the medical, fitness, and beauty professions. What is evolving today is a union of these varying disciplines.

Now, as we enter the new millennium, the world of beauty and health continues to change. Beauty and wellness integration is fast becoming the way of the world. It's what I like to call the inner route, or *home*. In taking the inner route—or coming home—I turned toward beauty and wellness practices designed for self-actualization—a more joyful, healthful, preventive approach to well-being. I plunged into energy healing and massage therapy training, along with training in yoga, herbalism, and aromatherapy. I learned transcendental meditation, went on a vision quest with Buster Yellow Kidney (the spiritual leader of the Blackfeet Indian Nation), performed yoga's early morning sun salutation on the edge of the Arabian Ocean, joined my sisters in a drumming circle, and went to regular trance (ecstatic) dance gatherings.

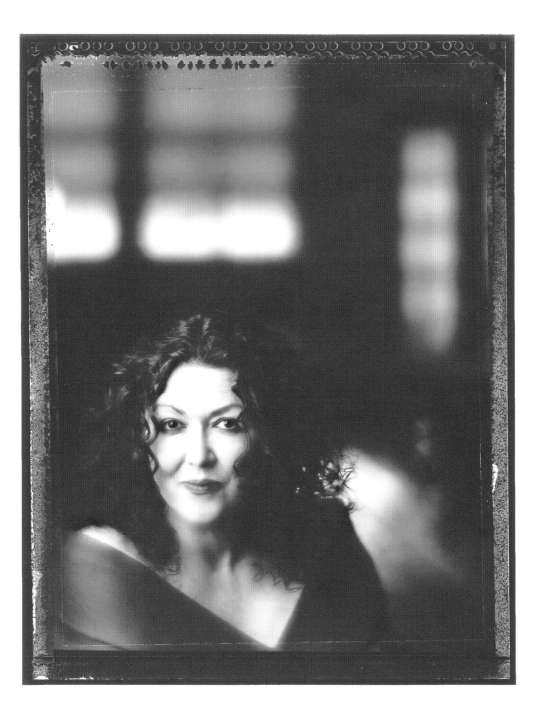

Coming home also meant tapping into and fully appreciating experiences I had as a child. Today, as an organic gardener, I truly appreciate having grown up on a farm. Farm life ingrained in me this pattern of striving toward finding harmony with the Earth. Growing up on the farm grounded me in the natural world of things—whether through the food we ate, the gardens we grew, or the animals we cared for. Growing up on the farm and feeling that nature surrounded and enveloped me in her comforting embrace was an incredible experience that lives on and is reflected in who I am today. I strive to bring the spirit of all these connections into every moment of every day because these were indeed joyful occasions of purity, naturalness, and innocence—in essence, love. Suffice it to say that when I left the farm, I embarked upon a journey of discovery.

I'm not exactly sure of the precise moment when all of my experiences came together and I woke up. It just sort of happened, and I found myself living and being on a whole new level. I became aware that the whole Earth was breathing, and I could feel the planet's pulse. This awakening to nature's rhythms allowed me to understand that God surrounds and permeates absolutely everything and everyone. This is the life force energy in all creation and us. This is the spirit of radiant beauty.

Today my company, The Janssen Source, Inc., provides resources to the beauty and wellness communities by creating multimedia programs as well as organizing and teaching beauty and wellness integration seminars and retreats. Yet even as I teach, write, produce, and direct, I continue to metamorphose, learning from some very powerful teachers, mentors, and students who shed light on my path.

Now it's my turn to shed a little light on *your* path. I hope you enjoy this book, which I liken to a nourishing meal. You can grant yourself time to digest and metabolize one chapter at a time, or, if you prefer, you can peruse the entire book at one sitting and nibble on only bits of information from a grand buffet.

So, there you have it. A brief introduction to *Radiant Beauty*, as well as its author. I hope that my work provides you with a sense of renewal, rejuvenation, and rebirth.

Mary Beth Janssen

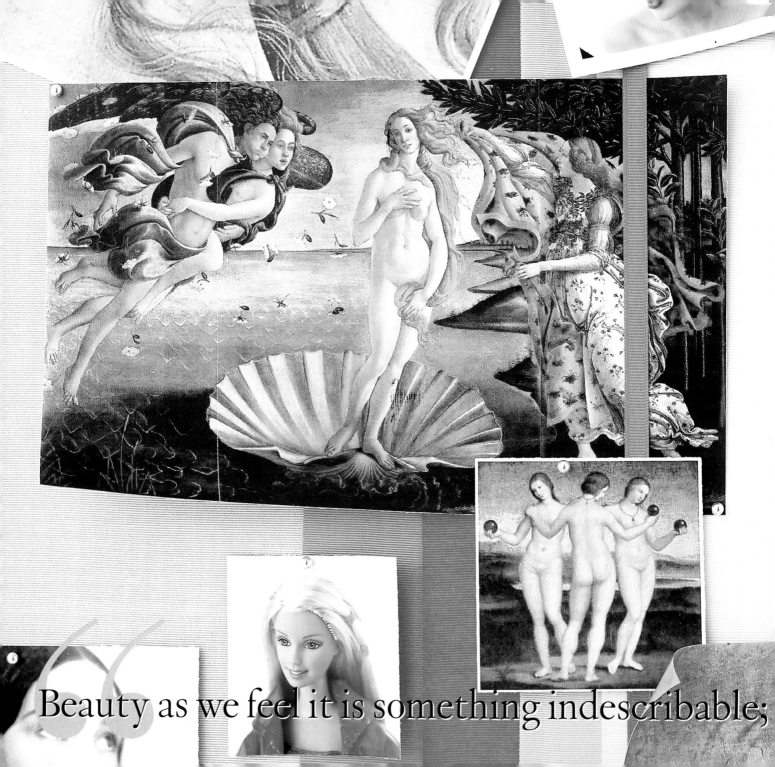

Beauty as we feel it is something indescribable;

beauty *defined*

what it is or what it means can never be said.

George Santayana

Organic **beauty** is the harmonious union of our external image with our internal sense of self. It is the art of being—everything that is life and style, grace and charm. It is my greatest wish that I can heighten your **awareness** of the beauty that you hold within, the beauty that you present to the world, and the beauty that surrounds you at all times. ● Some say beauty is so complex that it defies definition. Others claim that beauty is in the eye of the beholder, and individual **perceptions** define beauty—although these varying definitions may equal the number of people on Earth. Still others declare beauty to be something that comes in a box, an entity defined by the cosmetics and fashion industries. One thing is certain: Everyone has the ability to recognize beauty, whether with their eyes, their **soul**, or both. ● If we take the time to expand our awareness of beauty, we will find ourselves surrounded by it at every turn. Beauty will become something that pleases or satisfies not just the senses, but also the mind. We'll discover that **color**, form, texture, proportion, rhythmic motion, tone, and even behaviors or attitudes that create an emotional response are part of experiencing beauty. By appreciating beauty in every way it is expressed, we make life diverse, **joyful**, and meaningful.

" Whatever is in any way beautiful hath its source

Recognizing Our Own Beauty

When we use all our senses to recognize beauty—be it a caressing touch, a loving gaze, a fragrant aroma, an ethereal melody, or a succulent taste—we relate to beauty on a higher level of consciousness. This heightened awarenss epitomizes *organic* beauty. We begin to see beauty in absolutely anything, thus creating harmony and balance within the mind and body—a simply marvelous concept referred to as mind-body physiology. And let's not forget that an integral part of that harmony and balance includes the beauty within ourselves.

In this book, I challenge you to recognize and honor your own naked beauty. I realize that as you try raising your awareness and thus defining beauty in your own terms, you are simultaneously being bombarded by hundreds of outside influences. As you become more cognizant of these influences, however, you will find yourself able to work around them. Your new awareness will even void out some of these influences. When that happens, your own beauty will be free to shine. Then, as you begin reading the specifics of the organic beauty regimens in this book—treatments for skin, hair, nails, and so on—you will find yourself able to recognize, honor, and enhance your true, natural beauty.

Beauty Culture

People have sought beauty since time began, and it's fascinating how changing times and cultures alter how beauty is perceived. Exotic early Egyptian beauty rituals included everything from drawing intricate designs on the body with henna to coloring the eyelids with iridescent powder made from crushed beetles. Cleopatra softened her skin with sesame seed and barley packs and wore eyeliner made from crushed minerals. Some Roman beautifiers—now known to be extremely dangerous—included arsenic complexion wafers ingested to create lily white skin and toxic face powders made from metals such as sulfur, mercury, or lead. Wanting to appear sexually

# of beauty in itself, and is complete in itself...
Marcus Aurelius

aroused, women of the Italian Renaissance dilated their pupils with drops of belladonna. Despite the knowledge that blindness was a distinct possibility, women pursued this ritual in the name of beauty.

Sociocultural influences dictated these practices, just as modern culture and the media continue to influence our quest for beauty today. One can't help but wonder how the next millennium's civilization will view our current beauty ceremonies.

What Is Beauty Today?

In modern Westernized societies, the image of beauty can often be one that's superficially applied. I would like to suggest that we look back to ancient times, borrowing a bit of our ancestors' spiritual connection to beauty. This may mean adjusting your definition of beauty, moving away from superficial good looks as defined in the past by the beauty business and toward a balance of external and internal beauty. Holistically speaking, this balance brings us to a healthy, nurturing wholeness.

Outward beauty is but one part of organic beauty. The rest of the story hinges on inward beauty, which is an expression of balance and simplicity in one's life. When outward and inward beauty harmoniously coexist, our mind-body physiology exudes the most radiant beauty of all.

The Soul of Beauty

A holistic approach to personal care has been around for centuries, but it enjoyed a rebirth in the mid-1990s, when the spa culture became popular. People wanted to use natural, organic products at home, just as they did in spas. This interest in holistic products signaled a major step toward spiritual discovery. Suddenly beauty was not merely skin deep, but *soul* deep. Even the marketing world began putting soul in their advertisements. There were body cleansers that promised fulfillment,

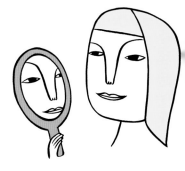

"There are as many kinds of beauty as there are

face moisturizers for stressed skin, cosmetics based on feng shui, and promises that we could exfoliate our way to enlightenment. These pledges and their meanings made an attractive package, and consumers bought both.

Although the beauty industry's message often proved more potent than its products, a few organic beauty products appeared that actually did adhere to holistic philosophies. Today there are many organic beauty products that contain certified organic ingredients and that are manufactured using processes that respect our natural environment. These are holistic products that enhance external beauty, internal wellness, and also the world around us. It is important, however, that we use these products only as a spark, to ignite internal good feelings while simultaneously enhancing external beauty.

An Image to Keep

In our image-based society, physical attractiveness is seen as a tremendous asset. This premise has been examined in numerous studies over the years, and one particularly insightful report comes from psychologist and researcher Nancy Etcoff in her book *Survival of the Prettiest: The Science of Beauty*. After considering Etcoff's book as well as many additional studies, several intriguing generalities came to light:

- Attractive people are perceived as friendlier.

- Better-looking students tend to do better in school, perhaps receiving more gratuitous guidance from their teachers.

- Mothers unconsciously give more attention to pretty babies.

- In relationships, the partner perceived as most attractive is more often the decision maker.

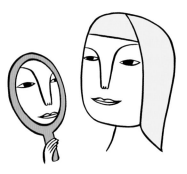

habitual ways of seeking happiness.
Charles Baudelaire

Perhaps we do judge a book by its cover!

So, by modern standards, what defines a "beautiful" person? An attractive face has been defined as symmetrical and of average proportions, with harmony in the placement and size of facial features. In several studies done by psychologists, women who were considered beautiful were found to have wide-set eyes, full lips, a smaller nose, and a petite chin. Extreme facial features are seen as off-putting. Studies have also shown that most people find the classic hourglass figure to be the most attractive body type for women.

Despite research, social mandates, and controlled studies, it still appears that the definition of beauty is fleeting. I've spent many years in the beauty business and have often been responsible for casting print and film models and actors, so I have seen firsthand how difficult it is to define beauty. For example, depending on the product being advertised and its target audience, requirements for a model can change dramatically. A particular model may be perfect for one product, but for another product she may not be blonde enough, exotic enough, slender enough, tall enough, or simply pretty enough.

Beauty Turns Quirky

Society's beauty standards change with the times. Unlike the 1950s or 1960s, parameters for today's beauty ideal have moved more toward the unique and unusual face. Many of the most popular fashion catalogs feature models with atypical beauty. Sometimes this includes a more ethnic or multicultural model, as well as more mature models.

Nowhere are our changing beauty standards more apparent than on television. I find it interesting that several of today's most successful television programs fall into the category of "reality

Is She Pretty Enough?

Our world is filled with people who judge themselves to be not pretty or handsome enough. Some of these people turn to unnatural and extreme methods, such as plastic surgery, to achieve their beauty ideal. Our culture of celebrity—movie stars, high-fashion models, sports figures—has created unrealistic expectations for many, particularly the young. This influence is vividly evident in the way young girls perceive their bodies. For example, more than two-thirds of a group of adolescent girls interviewed for a study published by *The Journal of Pediatrics* said magazine photos influenced their notion of how they should look, and 47 percent said they wanted to lose weight because of those pictures. Only 29 percent of the girls, however, were overweight by pediatric standards.

shows." I think this says something about our desire to connect with real people—people with imperfections. In some way, these shows validate the fact that it's okay to be less than perfect, creating a tidal wave of awareness in people's consciousness and flinging the door wide open to the premise of organic beauty.

Selling Beauty

Madison Avenue wields tremendous power over us, placing in our mind's eye the image of all we should desire, and thus feel we *need*. But just as the beauty industry uses us, we use the beauty industry, too. We use the products and services to create an image, bolster our self-esteem, and in essence cultivate beauty in the eye of the beholder *and* the beheld. If we achieve all this, we also optimize our feelings of power and attractiveness.

With an ever-changing menu of pleasing images and beauty products to choose from, it's wise to remember the saying "style over substance." I would like to propose a new spin on this old cliché: style combined with substance. If you are comfortable in your own skin and are inherently a compassionate, optimistic, and loving individual, aligning your sense of style with this profound inner knowledge of self is a powerful step toward enjoying a rich and fulfilling life. You will be innately beautiful above and beyond props, societally imposed standards, and surgeries.

Cultivating Beauty

If you consider the combined dollars spent on products and services, the United States beauty industry is a $50 billion–plus machine. Add the billions spent on weight loss endeavors, health clubs, and cosmetic surgeries, and you begin to fathom how deep our search reaches (not to mention how far our pockets stretch) in order to achieve beauty. In the United States, we spend more money on beauty than we do on education or social services!

Integrating Beauty

In this new millennium, health, nutrition, and quality of life are playing even greater roles in our interpretation of true beauty and fashion. And there's no doubt that real beauty begins with health. It is true health—feeling good inside and out—that allows beauty to emerge. Once you achieve true health, a cascade of benefits result, showing up as healthy hair, skin, and nails. In essence, the whole body becomes healthier. Achieving the balance of inner and outer health involves a holistic approach where you recognize the important connection between the body, mind, and spirit. It is when this wholeness—this connection—is disrupted that patterns of illness or disease may set in.

The word "health" is derived from the Old English word *hal*, meaning whole. Right from the start, "health" was seemingly intended to mean the condition of being whole in body, mind, and spirit. Putting it in slightly different words, we are the sum of what we eat, how we think, and what we do. If we eat poorly, smoke, take drugs, drink alcohol, forgo exercise, are pessimistic, are constantly stressed out, lack a sense of purpose, have toxic relationships in life, and lack spirituality, we are putting ourselves at greater risk for contracting disease. As everyone knows, disease wreaks havoc not only with our body's health, but also with our outward appearance—our natural beauty.

As the 21st century begins, we see a convergence of science and psychology, body and soul. There is even a relatively new hybrid science called psychoneuroimmunology, which studies the interaction between mind and body and how this relationship affects blood chemistry.

One example of this mind and body interaction is the effectiveness of positive affirmations, or good thoughts. It is scientifically proven that positive affirmations raise the immune system's white blood cell count. Amazing! What we believe and the way we act have a definite effect on our health. It is only logical to conclude, therefore, that our health changes and evolves according to our experiences and how we feel about those experiences.

Embracing Mindfulness

The Buddha was once asked, "What do you and your disciples practice?" He answered, "We sit, we walk, and we eat." The questioner was confused and asked, "Doesn't everyone sit, walk, and eat?" "Yes," replied the Buddha, "but when we sit, we know we are sitting. When we walk, we know we are walking. When we eat, we know we are eating."

This is the essence of mindfulness in our lives. Whether eating a meal, washing dishes, brushing your teeth, or making love, be mindful of every nuance of the experience. Understanding the moment gives you knowledge to make choices. You can embrace a moment because it is nurturing of health and beauty, or you can walk away because it depletes health and beauty. By enhancing and protecting the vitality of each moment, we learn how to reach our fullest potential and maintain ultimate health and beauty.

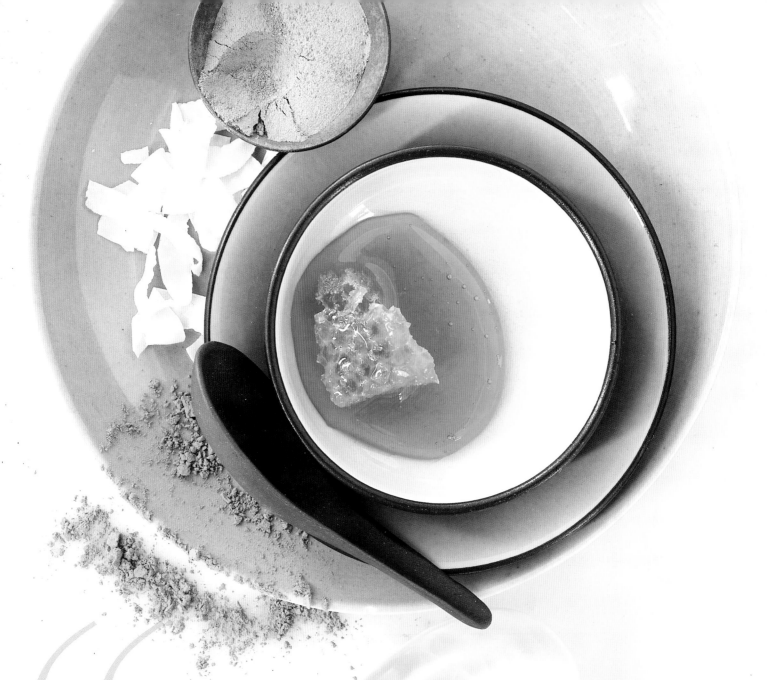

"Nature is fine in love, and where 'tis fine,

living *organically*

It sends some precious instance of itself.
William Shakespeare

We all want to taste life in its purest, most exalted form. This is the essence of **organic** and the essence of all that is beautiful. A deep understanding of what it means to be most vividly, most perfectly alive is intimately connected to an organic lifestyle, a **holistic** and ecological way of approaching life. If our thoughts and actions are organic in nature, we are respectful of and nourishing toward the sacredness of life. In respecting and nourishing the sacredness of life by organic means, we manifest beauty and health within the environment—an environment that includes us. ●

The time for organic is now—as an idea, a process, a **lifestyle**, and a state of being. The organic movement is growing stronger every year. When you join the organic tribe, you become part of an unprecedented trend toward a shift in awareness that is taking place worldwide. We are all questioning our **values**, asking "What are we doing to our environment, and in turn to our health?" While asking these questions, we are also seeking answers— solutions that help us feel good, realize exquisite health, and find an inner peace. These very solutions cannot help but lead to **true beauty**.

Organic Is Exploding!

People worldwide are striving to make their lifestyles more organic. Organic has gone mainstream, and it is no longer just about organic food. In the United States alone, organic product sales came in at approximately 6.6 billion during the year 2000. In 1989, the same marketplace pulled in only $78 million in sales. That's double-digit growth every year for over 10 years! This is clearly not a fad; it's global proof that people around the world feel very passionate about mind-body health and the health of our environment.

Organic is about the vibrant life force that is inherent in all of creation. My own definition of organic is somewhat malleable, exploring the philosophical, biological, scientific, as well as spiritual expressions of what it is to be organic. Some of you may define organic as produced without toxic chemical pesticides and nitrate-laden fertilizers, while others define organic as grown in harmony with the natural rhythms of the universe. Indeed, both definitions are correct. Whether referring to certified organic foodstuffs or natural, time-honored ingredients found in the wide variety of organic products in the marketplace, organic is about enhancing healthful living and beauty. Every organism on earth is influenced by the delicate ecosystem of which it is a part. Your body even has its own ecosystem! If this delicate ecosystem is compromised by toxins, whether physical, mental, or spiritual, the life force is being assaulted. Living organically is about waking up and remembering our wholeness. This enlightenment is quite profound and will forever change your world.

In the end, organic is about enhancing healthful living and beauty. To simplify matters, let's examine organic on its most basic level. The human body is not simply static matter, but rather vibrating energy. If we go to the deepest level, we are subatomic particles whirling around at lightning speed, on the verge of becoming matter. This fluctuation of energy and matter is life's cosmic dance. Seven million red blood cells blink in and out of existence in your body every second. Your pancreas regenerates virtually all of its cells every 24 hours. Your stomach lining is regenerated every 3 days, your

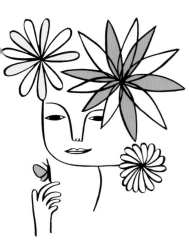

white blood cells every 10 days, and your brain protein every month. You shed 100,000 skin cells every minute! As you can see, your body is constantly working to regenerate itself. To successfully perform this renewal process, however, the human body needs nourishment in the form of optimal thought, food, and activity.

So, if we sense that changing our experiences would benefit our mind-body physiology, we should do it. Each person has the power to make choices that create balance and harmony in life. The good news is that changing our experiences sometimes means little more than changing our *perceptions* of those experiences! Throughout this book I will share simple ways in which you can reflect upon and enjoy your life experiences. By doing so, you'll be on the path to organic beauty.

Evolutionary Consciousness

Our thoughts, beliefs, feelings, and values deeply affect how we live. This is our consciousness guiding us. By exploring ways to live more consciously, we broaden the possibilities for peak experiences. This is all integral to living an organic lifestyle, a conscious and purposeful decision made from a heightened awareness that precipitates great positive changes.

For some, these changes will mean a reconnection with the natural world, and for others, they will mean maintaining an existing connection for a lifetime. From this connection come many more positive changes, resonating through the many parts of your life. After all, we are a part of nature, not separate from it. The environment is an extension of our mind-body physiology. We are recycled earth, water, and air—carbon, oxygen, hydrogen, nitrogen, and sulfur. We're made of the exact same stuff as all other living things. It is simply the configuration of our DNA that differentiates us.

Did You Know?

- According to The Environmental Working Group, a nonprofit environmental research organization, by the age of 5, millions of children have ingested up to 35 percent of a lifetime's worth of exposure to some carcinogenic pesticides.
- The Environmental Protection Agency considers 60 percent of all herbicides, 90 percent of all fungicides, and 30 percent of all insecticides to be potentially carcinogenic.
- The National Academy of Sciences estimates that pesticides are responsible for 20,000 cancer cases annually.
- The EPA estimates that 2.3 billion pounds of pesticides are applied annually to U.S. crops, lawns, gardens, parks, golf courses, and other lands.
- The National Cancer Institute found an increased risk of leukemia in children whose parents used pesticides in their homes or gardens.

"Man did not weave the web of life. He is merely a strand

Whatever we ingest from the earth becomes the tissues and organs that make up our bodies—the food we eat, the air we breathe, and the water we drink. Choosing an organic lifestyle nurtures balance and health within our own physiology, as well as that of the Earth.

Understanding the Cosmic Dance: The Rhythms of Nature

Sometimes it's easier to understand the importance of our connection to nature if we look at things on a more personal level. Circadian (24-hour), seasonal, tidal, and lunar rhythms synchronize every facet of your being. Together, these rhythms control the ebb and flow of your bodily functions—including sleep and wake cycles, body temperatures, hormonal levels, and menstrual cycles. To learn your own optimal time for waking, sleeping, eating, physical activity, and creativity, as well as for the elimination of toxins, you must tune in to nature's rhythms and to the valuable sensations and intuition within yourself.

Working the night shift, taking a transcontinental flight, or eating a large meal before bed can throw your biological rhythms off balance. When these body rhythms go off track, dysfunction can result, including exhaustion, poor physical health, weak emotional health, and a general malaise that dims your natural beauty. Now let's go back to that grander level: When the natural rhythms of our planet are disrupted, our environment or nature shifts into an imbalance—not unlike the imbalance that can affect the human body.

Cooperating with Nature

In agriculture as well as gardening, the word organic refers to an Earth-friendly process of planting, growing, harvesting, and processing plants for food, fiber, and medicine, as well as for household and personal-care items. The term organic means that a plant or the ingredients within a product have been grown in biologically rich soil without the use of toxic chemical pesticides and fertilizers, in a way that supports the Earth, its

in it. Whatever he does to the web, he does to himself.

Chief Seattle

ecosystems, and the inherent balance within nature. By rotating crops between fields, using compost, and planting cover crops such as rye, oats, alfalfa, or hairy vetch, the organic farmer nourishes the soil and greatly reduces plant pests. These cover crops will be tilled into the earth before the regular growing season begins, creating a rich mixture of minerals and decomposing plant matter that serves as food for the incredible amount of microorganisms, fungi, and earthworms found in the unique ecosystem.

Everything the organic farmer does flows from a great deal of forethought, genuine passion, and a commitment to Mother Earth and her environment. To go full circle, building organic soil in this manner encourages tremendous sustainability and biodiversity, which will enable organic farmers to continuously bring us the wonderful organic plants used to create organic food and beauty products.

Certified Organic Provides the Standard

Stringent certification procedures are in place worldwide by which organic farmers, gardeners, and processors become certified and in turn bring certified organic products to the marketplace. In the United States, all certification is under the jurisdiction of the United States Department of Agriculture as set forth by the National Organic Standards Board. Look for the USDA Certified Organic label.

Certified organic food, whether from a plant or an animal, contains no genetically engineered organisms, and it was not irradiated to exterminate bacteria. In addition, certified organic food that originated from a living animal has been produced in a way that respects life—both that of the human eating the food and that of the animal being used for food. While being raised, these animals were fed only certified organic feed and were not exposed to high levels of growth hormones and antibiotics. On a more spiritual level, organically raised animals roam the pastures, take in fresh air, enjoy a bit of sunlight, and in essence have a life. The more you expose yourself to organic foods, produced from plants or animals, the healthier your entire body will be.

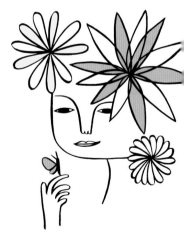

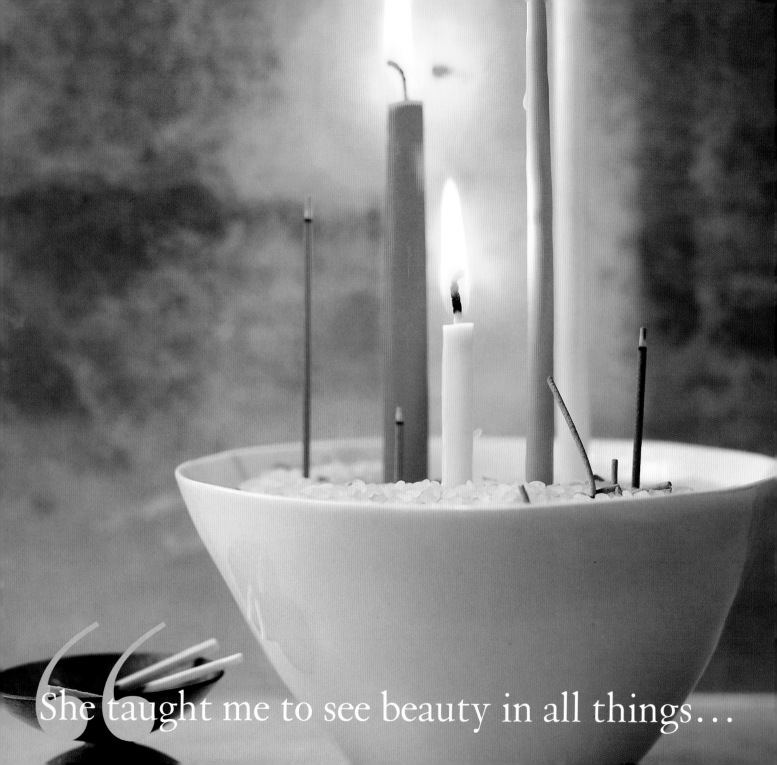

She taught me to see beauty in all things…

the spirit of *organic beauty*

that inside each thing a spirit lived...

Maria Campbell

Spirit is the **life force** within the universe, the Earth, and all beings. In order to experience spirit, you must first recognize that there is no duality—separation—between the mind and the physical body. Once you understand this, you can realize the **ecstasy** in your own mind-body physiology, which is the heart and soul of organic beauty. Making this connection is the surest way to uncover your true beauty. ● Any consciousness-expanding approach that helps us slow down and quiet our "monkey mind" will release negative **energy** and promote awareness of spirit, creating organic beauty—beauty from the inside out and the outside in. This allows a person's unique **aura** to shine, making it apparent to you as well as others through your heightened vitality, manner of speech, **elegance** in posture, and grace of movement. You begin to see clearly everything that the mind-body physiology does. Try it! Observe yourself reading this book right now. Stay with this observation as long as you can. Once you begin to really **share** your own experiences with yourself, it will become clear where, when, and how a behavior or attitude compromises your health and beauty. Conversely, you will begin to identify and perpetuate those experiences that **enhance** your true beauty.

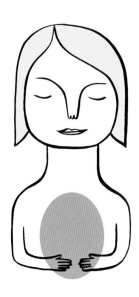

Witnessing

To consciously observe how your mind-body physiology experiences life is called witnessing. This concept is about as organic as you can get. By witnessing, you watch yourself make choices with and directed toward your spirit, rather than because of physical needs or learned habits. For example, consider how you wake up. Do you bolt out of bed and stumble to the shower, barely aware of the time, date, or century? To witness your own morning and nurture your life force, wake up slowly. Make arising each morning a delightful ritual.

Stretch. Do you do yoga? If not, I highly recommend you try it.

Enjoy a moment of meditation. This may be a brief moment for prayer, a few minutes of complete silence and inner peace, time to ponder the day ahead, or perhaps a brief respite when you give thanks for all that is about to happen.

Practice self-massage. Use organic almond oil and a few drops of rosemary and lavender essential oils to enliven your skin.

Step into the shower. Awaken and cleanse yourself with an organic bodywash.

As you move through the day, greet people in a nonjudgmental and compassionate way. Express gratitude for every facet of the beauty that surrounds you. In order to celebrate life in such a broad, unprejudiced manner, many of us first may need to consider a little emotional cleansing and a few changes in our attitudes.

Housecleaning

Letting your emotions control your life creates tremendous stress. It's important to understand that much of the stress we feel is relative to our perception of a given situation. When you learn how to change your perceptions of or emotional attitudes toward stressful situations, you remove their ability to negatively affect you. This is a

"No one can make you feel inferior without your

powerful step toward creating the harmonious balance that brings emotional well-being as well as exquisite beauty. It also makes room for your smile—and what's more attractive than a vibrant laugh or a dazzling smile?

To begin the cleansing process, try observing your emotions. Begin simply, looking at one emotion toward one situation.

Identify the sensations that the emotion creates in your body.
Verbalize or write down how the emotion makes you feel.
Release the emotion and celebrate this release. Now this negative emotion no longer controls you, but you control it!

If this technique seems overwhelming, ask a friend or loved one for support. Or, you may want to consider professional help. Talking to someone removed from your stressful situation can bring tremendous relief, renewal, and even rebirth.

If you neglect the occasional emotional cleansing and instead crawl into a shell, you risk becoming anesthetized. Before you know it, you've gone a lifetime without experiencing pure, unadulterated joy. Make a conscious decision to stay awake, alive, and engaged in every facet of life.

Next Stop: Compassion

I'm very fortunate to work with Dr. Deepak Chopra, and I've been tremendously inspired by him. Dr. Chopra says, "We are all doing the very best that we can from the level of consciousness that we're in." This one statement rocks my world!

When you try to understand where someone is coming from, you automatically become less judgmental. When you become less

Jump In!

Connecting with spirit is an endless journey, and it's often one that takes you little farther than your front door. Realize that this path includes grand accomplishments and also the tiniest of things. It means that anything that allows us to feel the life force flowing effortlessly through our bodies nurtures our soul, strengthens our self-esteem, and helps us regain all the grand passion that is our birthright. To help you find your own unique way to connect with spirit, try any one of the approaches described in this chapter. What I can simply say is, "Jump right in, the water is mighty fine."

consent.
Eleanor Roosevelt

judgmental, you become more tolerant. When you become more tolerant, you are more able to forgive. And when you are able to forgive, you have the capacity to love unconditionally. Compassion creates a remarkable chain of positive energy that results in the most radiant beauty of all.

Defusing Stress

Personal stress is defined as the inability to cope with a real or imagined threat to your well-being, resulting in a series of responses and adaptations by the mind and body. It's estimated that approximately 80 percent of all visits to a primary care physician stem from stress-related issues. That's all the more reason to witness everything you do, change your attitudes, and perform the spiritual practice of compassion. Commit to living mindfully instead of mindlessly, and look at everything you do as sacred and organic. Learn to calm down. If stress is permitted to hum along unabated, serious consequences can result. Think about it: What does stress do to you? It is essential that you identify the negative stressors in your life and discover ways to counter them.

A Beautiful Balance

So how do we find balance—and thus spirit—in our often-busy lives? There are so many wonderful techniques you can try, including breathing techniques, meditation, and yoga. Sensory modulation through nutritional, herbal, massage, and aroma therapies can help as well. Naturally, a healthy amount of physical activity also figures into the equation. In short, adjusting what you take in through your senses can assist in pacifying a wide range of stressful emotions, including anxiety, anger, and depression, to name only a few.

Let's look at several consciousness-raising approaches that help calm the mind-body physiology and thus place that vital connection with spirit within your grasp.

Breathwork

Breath is synonymous with spirit and life. When you inhale, you take in air molecules that oxygenate your blood and send it coursing through your veins to every cell in your body. Every breath you exhale sends carbon dioxide into the environment, making the grass grow greener. Breathing naturally creates a kind of internal rhythm that keeps your organs and systems functioning in physiological harmony. It sounds simple enough, yet you would be amazed at how many people's breathing is less than optimal.

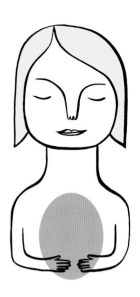

To understand correct breathing, watch a sleeping baby. The baby's abdomen rises and falls with each breath because he's using his diaphragm—the broad muscle sandwiched between the lungs and the abdominal area. Adults tend to unconsciously hold the diaphragm frozen. Check your breathing right now. Put one hand on your chest and one on your abdomen. Inhale and exhale. You want your abdomen to extend outward as you bring in a deep breath and contract inward as you exhale. This is diaphragmatic breathing.

When done properly, diaphragmatic breathing brings air down into the lower portion of the lungs, where the oxygen exchange is most efficient. The physiological effects are tremendous. The heart rate slows, blood pressure decreases, digestion improves, muscles relax, anxiety eases up, and the mind calms down. Anyone can use breathing to develop better sleep patterns, improve blood circulation, and increase their mindfulness. In one study, diaphragmatic breathing reduced the frequency of hot flashes in menopausal woman by 50 percent. Breathwork can also help those overcoming addictions.

A Simple Breathing Exercise

Do the following exercise often, and hopefully you will make diaphragmatic breathing an unconscious effort. You can try it sitting up straight or lying down, preferably in a quiet place where no one will disturb you. If you like, place a hand on your abdomen while you do it.

> # " The quieter you become, the more you can hear.
> *Ram Dass*

Bring in a deep breath through your nose. Feel the warm air flowing into the deepest recesses of your lungs.

Visualize the energy from this breath flowing to every part of your body.

Feel your muscles relax. Your abdomen should expand outward.

Slowly exhale through your nose. Your abdomen will move inward. As your breath flows outward, visualize any stress you feel dissolving away.

Creative Visualization

While witnessing connects you to the real moment, visualization (or imagery) takes you to where you would like to be. Visualization is a method used to form desirable images in the mind, like a beautiful scene at a relaxing place. In your mind, you want to become very intimate with every detail of this place. Use all of your senses. Experience the colors, aromas, textures, and sounds. Feel the movement of air. Remember to breathe deeply and rhythmically! Stay with this visualization for at least 5 to 10 minutes.

Once you get the hang of visualization, you will find it a very powerful technique for programming your subconscious to enhance your beauty. Visualize your body strong and toned. Visualize your skin smooth and glowing. Visualize your eyes vibrant, clear, and dazzling. You may manifest what you visualize!

Repeat this breathing technique 10 times for quick relaxation, or more times for greater effect. Many variations exist for heightening the experience, from prolonging each inhalation and exhalation to extending your overall practice length. You may count during each inhalation and exhalation, perhaps to five. (This can be adjusted according to your lung capacity.) You can also combine your breathing with more advanced visualization to accentuate relaxation. Imagine breathing in the ocean air, the scent of flowers, or whatever aroma brings you peace. Try deep diaphragmatic breathing at least two or three times a day.

Meditation

Meditation has been and remains an integral part of the world's spiritual traditions, and in it we find great richness, depth, and mysticism. When done mindfully, meditation can alter your perception of things, making the big things seem very small. You'll find yourself becoming more emotionally flexible and accepting. Along with my daily breathing practice, meditation helps me reduce stress and find peace. I highly recommend it to you.

Meditation in Practice

Ideally, you want to make meditation a daily ritual, since its most profound results are seen if you practice it for 20 to 30 minutes twice each day. The best meditation times are dusk and dawn, when the vibrations of our circadian rhythms are most calm and peaceful.

Choose a regular, quiet place to meditate. Make this place special—light a candle, burn incense, or create an altar if you wish.

Use a personal mantra, a chosen word (Om, peace, love, your name, and so on), or a chant. If you prefer, simply become aware of your breath by doing a few minutes of diaphragmatic breathing, either alone or coupled with yoga postures to calm and center yourself before beginning.

Sit in a chair with your spine as straight as possible. You may also sit on the floor in the cross-legged lotus position. Yoginis, or yoga practitioners, refer to this as the easy sitting position. If you need back support, sit against a rolled towel or cushion.

Close your eyes and shift your attention to your breathing. Breathe deeply, smoothly, and naturally. Pay attention to the flow of your breath as you inhale and exhale. Do not try to alter or control your breath. If you are distracted by thoughts, sounds in the surrounding environment, or sensations in the body, let them come and go as you bring your attention back to your breathing.

Continue this process for 20 to 30 minutes. Slowly and gently open your eyes. Bring your awareness back to your surroundings.

Don't worry about whether you're doing this right. Show up with the intention to meditate, and you've already reaped a measure of the benefit that this practice will bring.

Consciousness in Motion

Every minute you devote to exercise is a blessing for your body, mind, and soul. Physical activity is vital to our well-being, and it is one of the most powerful beautifiers. Bodies love to move and be active, whether for work, dance, or just pure enjoyment.

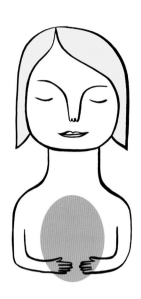

We're Heavyweights

The Surgeon General tells us that only 26 percent of the United States population exercises regularly. If you're not in that percentage, the big question is how to inspire yourself to become active. Try using your visualization skills to imagine yourself exercising through the various stages of life before you. Perhaps you can visualize yourself at 75, surfing the waves, tooling around town on a bike, or running 5 miles each morning. See and feel how healthy, vital, and filled with energy you are, still enjoying every moment of every day. A word of caution, though: Anyone whose body is not used to physical activity should first check in with his or her primary care physician. With this expert's blessing, visualize yourself beginning slowly but powerfully, get off the couch, and then get moving!

If visualization can't get you moving, maybe a few facts will.

● Physical activity benefits your musculoskeletal system, heart and blood vessels, bodily processes, mental processes, and longevity. This is largely a result of improved cardiovascular and respiratory functioning, which enhances the transport of oxygen and nutrients to every cell in your body.

● Physical activity enhances the movement of carbon dioxide and waste products from the tissues of the body into the bloodstream and into the eliminative organs. These combined actions improve your energy levels, stamina, and ability to handle stress.

● Those who exercise regularly tend to have higher self-esteem and are generally happier.

● As for outer beauty, the more efficient your blood circulation is, the more beautiful your skin, hair, nails, and eyes will be.

"Health is the second blessing that we mortals are

Let's Get Physical

Physical activity includes cardiovascular, flexibility, and strengthening activities. Try to create a balance of these three types in your daily routine.

Cardiovascular or aerobic activity reduces stress and enhances your heart health, immune system, endurance, longevity, and overall quality of life. For every 1 hour of aerobic activity, there may be a 2-hour increase in longevity. Consider brisk walking, jogging, swimming, biking, dancing, and power yoga.

Flexibility exercises are great for easing physical tension, improving your range of motion, improving your agility, and helping you connect body, mind, and spirit. Concentrating on your breath during these activities brings you face to face with your energy source. Try yoga or tai chi.

Strengthening or weight-bearing activities enhance your power, endurance, and coordination. Along with aesthetic benefits, your body will also burn fat more efficiently. You may choose to use either free weights or machines, as well as performing weight-bearing activities such as walking, yoga, or Pilates.

Yoga

You may have noticed that yoga showed up in all three categories of physical activity. The intensity or gentleness, along with the flow of your yoga practice, determines the benefits. For many, yoga is a new and inspiring physical activity, but it has actually been around for over 5,000 years! Yoga, an ancient Hindu practice, means union or yoke and can be a complete philosophy for living. It can weave your mind, body, and spirit together in a mutually supportive relationship. Calming yet invigorating, yoga postures, or asanas, when coupled with mindful breathing, can make you stronger and more flexible, while also raising your consciousness. I encourage you to take a class, check your cable television listings, or look into the many instructional tapes and videos available.

Love the One You Are

Any consciousness-raising approach where you are exercising from the inside out and the outside in can help you calm the mind-boy physiology and thus connect with your spirit. While you're exercising your mind and body, remember to stay with reality! Recognize that each one of us is born with a particular body shape. Don't try to conform to the fantasy bodies of professional models. Neither visualization nor physical activity can change the limits of reality. Both practices can, however, help you become the absolute best you can be.

capable of, a blessing that money cannot buy.

Izaak Walton

" And in her cheeks the vermeil red did

the nature of *skin*

shew, Like roses in a bed of lilies shed…
Edmund Spenser

Let's look at skin in its unabashed **nakedness**. Your skin is your body's largest organ, weighing anywhere from 6 to 12 pounds. Always very busy, your **skin** sheds over 1 million cells every hour. A single square centimeter of skin contains 200 nerve endings, 100 sweat glands, 15 oil glands, 10 hairs, 2 cold receptors, and 25 pressure-sensing receptors. ● It shields you from rain, snow, and sunshine, and it protects you with a constant bath of moisture and natural oils. It breathes in **oxygen** and expels carbon dioxide, is a primary organ for excreting toxins, and regulates your body temperature. It is also involved in the metabolism and storage of fat. When exposed to sunlight, it produces the **life-essential** vitamin D. ● Truly, skin connects us with life, since it is through our skin that we begin the experience of touch. Think of all the **sensations** your skin allows you to delight in, whether through touching or being touched. Deep inside our bodies, without our even being aware of it, the mere action of stroking one's skin releases a flood of natural **feel-good** chemicals. The gamut of life's experiences is projected onto and deep within your skin's surface. This and so much more is your skin. How is your skin feeling today?

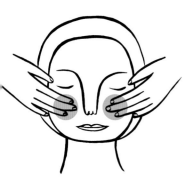

Skin Anatomy 101

For just a minute, let's talk about your skin's anatomy. This will help you create a balanced skin-care regimen and ultimately maintain healthy, youthful-looking skin. Your skin has three layers: the epidermis, the dermis, and the subcutaneous layer. Each layer has its own function and needs.

The epidermis is the outermost layer. This is the layer containing melanin, which gives our skin its color. The epidermis is the first place you will see positive results from a regular skin-care regimen. Deeper epidermal skin cells are alive and reproducing, but by the time these cells reach the outermost layer of your epidermis, they have keratinized, or died. These dead cells, when combined with your skin's secretions of sebum and perspiration, waterproof your skin. To avoid dull, dry skin and clogged pores, it is essential that these cells be continuously sloughed off.

The dermis consists of connective tissue containing a portion of your skin's blood supply, lymph channels, nerve endings, sebaceous and sweat glands, and hair follicles. This connective tissue is made up mainly of collagen and elastic fibers (both proteins), and it provides elasticity, firmness, and strength. When neglected, sagging and wrinkles may result. Beyond neglect, the dermis also naturally begins to sag and wrinkle as we age. A primary focus of your skin-care routine should be to nourish and protect this layer, but I urge you to be leery of any over-the-counter products that claim to restore the dermis. Ingredients in nonprescription products cannot penetrate to the dermis because penetration would by definition qualify these products as medicinal. The best way to protect the dermis is to wear a sunblock with SPF 15 or higher anytime you go outdoors.

The subcutaneous layer, a fatty layer primarily made of adipose tissue, lies beneath the dermis. The subcutaneous layer also holds a portion of your skin's blood supply. This layer protects our internal organs and provides insulation. Essential fatty acids (good oils) feed and lubricate this layer. To make sure you get enough of these good oils, take 1 to 2 tablespoons of flaxseed oil daily, along with at least two 500 milligram capsules daily of borage or evening primrose oil. Your skin and hair will benefit.

Throughout this chapter, I'll be mentioning these five basic techniques for skin care.

1. Cleansing. Washing skin with a gentle cleansing agent to remove dirt and oil and to balance the skin.

2. Toning. Applying a clarifying liquid to firm and stimulate skin tissue, reduce pore size, and remove cleanser residue.

3. Moisturizing. Applying hydrating lotions or creams that are humectant (drawing moisture into the skin), emollient (preserving moisture already existing in the skin), and lubricating (laying a protective layer on the outside of the skin).

4. Exfoliating. Removing the top, dead layers of skin cells and debris to encourage better cell turnover and to prevent clogged pores.

5. Protecting. Adhering to the above four techniques ultimately results in the vital protection our skin needs—protection that encourages healthy skin-cell turnover; safeguards skin's natural acid mantle; and helps maintain skin's natural strength, elasticity, and resiliency.

Protecting the Skin Barrier

The most important goals in organic skin care are to encourage the rapid turnover of skin cells and to maintain the skin's natural acid mantle, which is a combination of sebum and perspiration that your body secretes to moisturize your skin's surface. Achieving these goals will help rebuild damaged collagen and elastin (the chief protein in your skin's elastic fibers) in order to maintain skin strength, elasticity, and resiliency.

In this chapter, we'll cover several important methods that optimize cellular turnover—from the inside out, as well as from the outside in. One method involves using deep-cleansing masks and alpha and beta hydroxy acids to help maintain efficient skin-cell turnover. These natural organic fruit acids exfoliate dead surface cells. And

Gammy used to say, 'Too much scrubbing takes

unlike chemical peels given by some dermatologists, AHAs don't penetrate beyond the epidermis and thus are much gentler to your skin.

To protect your skin's acid mantle, which covers your entire body, use gentle, acid-balanced cleansers to wash your skin. Avoid antibacterial or deodorant soaps, which tend to be harsh.

Why Organic Skin Care?

When we're young, our body is programmed to maintain clear, smooth, soft skin, and we have to really ignore our skin or take it for granted to derail this program. As we age, however, our skin begins to work less efficiently, thinning out, losing elasticity, and sagging. Exposure to stress—environmental, physical, or mental—only exacerbates this natural aging process. And mind you, when I talk about aging skin I don't mean 50- or 60-year-old skin. These changes can begin at a much younger age if your skin does not receive proper care.

Proper care does *not* have to mean using lots of expensive and complicated products. What I'm referring to is organic skin care, a logical and relatively simple approach that holistically nurtures your skin's natural ability to maintain good health. It is about therapies that treat our skin from the inside out and from the outside in.

What Condition Is Your Skin In?

Skin is generally classified as normal or healthy, dry, oily, combination, sensitive/irritated, or mature (which may connote a variety of conditions, including dry and flaky, oily, acne-prone, or sensitive). Some experts question whether normal skin even exists these days, given our exposure to physical, emotional, and environmental

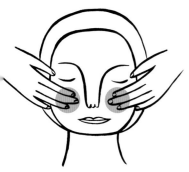

the life right out of things.'

toxins. In addition, it's important to remember that your skin classification is as variable as the seasons and your age, menstrual cycles, medication intake, environmental influences, and lifestyle choices. Therefore your skin type is always in transition. What's normal today may be oily tomorrow. Because of this, you need to be mindful and adapt your skin-care regimen accordingly.

Normal Skin

The most important aspect of caring for normal skin is to diligently work toward keeping it normal—maintenance, maintenance, maintenance! A regimen for this skin type should not strip natural oils and moisture or compromise the protective skin barrier in any way.

Dry Skin

A dull, sometimes flaky appearance and a rough, coarse, tight, and possibly itchy feel are characteristics of dry skin. This type of skin needs moisture or oil to keep it pliable and healthy. Moisturizers that are humectant (having an ability to attract and retain moisture) and emollient (having an ability to inhibit the loss of moisture and therefore have a softening and smoothing effect) are most effective in drawing moisture toward the skin's surface and holding it there to plump and moisturize the outer epidermal layer. To best treat and nourish dry skin, here are a few suggestions.

● Stop using antibacterial and deodorant soaps. They are drying, and they create an imbalance in our skin flora. In addition, research studies found that constant use of antibacterial soaps is helping to create new forms of antibiotic-resistant bacteria.

● When you bathe, cut back on the amount of time you spend in the shower or bath, use tepid to warm water, and thoroughly rinse off all cleansers. Consider splashing your face with cool water (preferably filtered water, purified through a showerhead or sink faucet filter attachment) in the morning, followed by a gentle, hydrating toner, and then a moisturizer.

● Use organic towels (those made from 100 percent organically grown cotton) and washcloths with a gentle touch. When drying off, blot or pat your skin until it's barely damp, then apply moisturizer. Applying moisturizer over damp skin acts to trap and hold more moisture in the skin.

● Drink burdock tea to cleanse the blood. Sweeten your tea with a bit of licorice root or stevia. Do this several times a day for one week and repeat every few months. This practice is particularly good for your blood circulation (cleansing and detoxifying the blood), and anything done for the blood helps bring more nutrients to your skin.

Get Naked

Get a healthy dose of nakedness every day. Go face to face with your skin. Sleep naked, drink your morning coffee in the buff, give yourself a full body massage with an organic plant oil like sweet almond oil before taking a shower. Feel your skin and the underlying tissues. Here's the naked truth: Getting comfortable with your own nudity not only provides great pleasure, but also allows you to recognize changes in your skin—changes that might require medical attention. What are you waiting for? Go get comfortable with the skin you're in.

Oily Skin

Oil or sebum excreted from the sebaceous glands help keep your skin lubricated and carry dead surface skin cells away. Oily skin does all this in overabundance, and while this skin type tends to be genetic, lifestyle choices—poor nourishment, improper skin care, excessive stress—may worsen the situation. Scrupulous yet gentle skin care is required to ensure that all this extra oil does not close off pore openings, clogging them and potentially lead to acne. Here are several of my favorite organic treatments for oily skin.

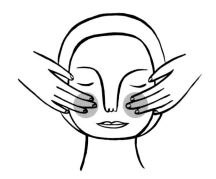

● Use a mild cleanser with warm water. Hot water and harsh cleansers only throw your skin into a tailspin!

● Avoid getting hair-care products on your face, or at least thoroughly wash off any products that hit your skin. If you neglect a complete rinsing, you may end up blocking your skin's pores.

● Use skin-care formulas and cosmetics that are water-based and noncomedogenic (products that will not clog your pores).

● Always remove makeup before bed.

● Watch your diet. A well-balanced, organic, whole foods diet will do more for your skin than any over-the-counter product could hope to accomplish.

● Chill out! The body produces more androgen hormones when stressed, and these hormones stimulate sebaceous glands to pump out more sebum.

Combination Skin

As you assess your face and body skin, you may see that you have a combination of skin types. This requires different treatments in different areas or alternating treatments during the week. For example, if you have an oily t-zone through the forehead, nose, and mouth area and normal or dry skin on the remainder of your face, apply a clay-based mask in the oily area and a creamy moisturizing mask in the dry area. (For more information on masks, see "Natural Masks and Exfoliants" on page 50.) In addition to using the right combination of treatments, look for products that contain balancing herbs or essential oils like calendula, chamomile, and lavender.

Sensitive and Mature Skin Types

Gentle products and treatments are essential for sensitive and mature skin types. These skin types benefit from a balancing massage of cooling plant and essential oils combined. Since neither skin type responds well to chemical peels, you might want to try a mild fruit acid and enzyme peel that helps gently shed the outside layer of dead skin, instead.

Coping with Acne

If you suffer from acne, I recommend that you see an experienced skin-care professional. Some causes and solutions for acne fall specifically into a medical doctor's domain. Treatment for acne should be gentle and consistent with high-quality organic skin-care products. I use tea tree essential oil when I feel an eruption coming on. Simply put a bit of this oil, available at health or whole foods stores, on an organic cotton swab and dab it onto the problem area. Do not rinse off. Or try a purchased or homemade toner made of peppermint or lemon essential oils, and mist your skin with it throughout the day. To make a toner, add 3 to 5 drops of the essential oil to 8 ounces of water, shake thoroughly, and let the mixture sit for 24 hours. Strain it through an organic paper coffee filter, pour the mix into a clean spray bottle, and spritz your face after cleansing or to simply freshen the skin. If you have oily skin, check organic product labels for the following ingredients: calendula, chamomile, sage, vitamins A (beta carotene), C, and E, and yarrow.

For women approaching or experiencing menopause, it seems that estrogen supplements increase your skin's thickness, moisture content, and amount of collagen fibers, while decreasing wrinkle depth and pore size. I am not suggesting hormone replacement therapy as a solution to aging skin, but I am suggesting that you research natural hormonal replacement therapies with your physician or another qualified person. Many fine options exist today. There are also many state-of-the-art skin-care products that address aging skin and its response to natural hormone depletion. When seeking out some of these skin-care products, check the product labels for one or more of the following ingredients, all prized for their effect on mature skin: DHEA, Ester-C, alpha lipoic acid, hemp seed oil, chamomile, liposomes, vitamin A (beta carotene), vitamin C, and vitamin E.

Secrets for Healthy Skin

Healthy skin is alive with vibrating energy. It is radiant, smooth, supple, elastic, and moist. It also has a slight flush to it from optimal blood circulation. Antioxidants are hard at work, hormones are balanced, and stress is under control. Oil and sweat glands are intelligently and lovingly bathing your skin with just the right amount of natural oil and moisture, which in turn maintains the skin's natural acid mantle. All the while, healthy, youthful skin is experiencing a constant state of renewal, turning over and shedding skin cells in a sort of healthful internal dance. Every cell in your body is communicating and working harmoniously. This is synergy in motion.

While this wonderful balance is indeed how your skin wants to react, you can damage this balance by putting your skin in harm's way. You can, however, avoid much external damage by thinking about everything you do. This is sometimes easier said than done, since many people don't even realize that routine activities are damaging their skin. Here are a few perfectly natural ways to create beautiful skin.

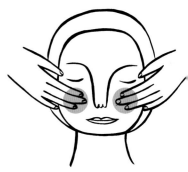

Reduce Stress

When you encounter extreme stress, your body tends to naturally divert an extra amount of nourishing blood to your internal organs. This is part of the "fight or flight" response, and a true protective measure for your heart, kidneys, and liver. At the same time, however, this phenomenon robs your skin of its nourishing blood supply and wreaks havoc with your skin's appearance. Stress can also depress your immune system, leaving your skin easy prey for viruses that cause cold sores, shingles, and other ailments. To rebalance and protect your skin, you want to control stress. Remember, wherever a thought goes, a molecule goes. Visualize beautiful skin. Meditate, breathe deeply, dance, or do whatever it takes to relax and invigorate yourself. In this way, you will calm your hormones and ultimately make a huge difference in the condition of your skin—particularly when it comes to acne.

Eat Right

A varied diet of organic whole foods, rich with a balance of proteins, carbohydrates, monounsaturated fats, and natural antioxidants, provides all the necessary daily requirements to generate healthy skin. We need the protein for skin growth and regeneration. We need the supply of antioxidants in a balanced diet to stave off free-radical damage. You can also do your skin a world of good by reducing your saturated animal fat intake and avoiding artificial ingredients and chemical pollutants.

Calcium. Found in dairy products, broccoli, cauliflower, and beans (including adzuki, almonds, soy, and pinto).

Essential fatty acids. Found in fish, flaxseed, and flaxseed oils.

Folic acid. Found in green leafy vegetables (like beet greens, chard, kale, and spinach), bean sprouts, legumes, peanuts, wheat germ, and yeast.

Iron. Found in apricots, brown rice, cereal (like granola), green vegetables, millet, oats, organ meats (like liver), red meat, raisins, wheat, and wholegrain bread.

Magnesium. Found in avocados, dark green vegetables, dried apricots, fish, fresh nuts and seeds (like sesame and pumpkin seeds), soy foods, and whole grains.

Protein. Found in dairy products, grains, legumes, meat, nuts and seeds, and soy foods.

Selenium. Found in brazil nuts, brewers yeast, garlic, liver, onions, shellfish, wheat germ, and whole grains.

Vitamin A. Found in red and yellow fruits and vegetables (like carrots, peaches, and pumpkins); green vegetables (like broccoli); and dark, leafy vegetables; eggs; hard cheese; and liver.

Vitamin B complex. Found in avocados, blackstrap molasses, brewers yeast, chicken, collards, fish, green vegetables, kale, liver, potatoes, soybeans, and whole grains.

Vitamin B$_{12}$. Found in chicken, cottage cheese, eggs, haddock, halibut, liver, tuna, and yogurt.

Vitamin C. Found in broccoli, citrus fruits, kiwi, peppers, regular and sweet potatoes, strawberries, and watermelon.

Vitamin E. Found in avocados, cold pressed wheat germ oil and safflower oil, eggs, green vegetables, and oily fish (like salmon and mackerel).

Zinc. Found in asparagus, eggs, endive, lobster (and other shellfish), mushrooms, mussels, oysters, pumpkinseeds, pecans, radishes, turkey, and whole grains.

"Let the beauty we love be what we do.

Rumi

I could go on and on about nutrition, but that would probably make this book too heavy to lift! So I'll simply say that good nutrition is absolutely vital to beautiful skin. Diet affects every part of your body, and when one part of you fails to function properly, residual effects eventually impact your skin. For more information on progressive approaches to nutrition, see "Recommended Reading and Resources" on page 134.

Practice Sun Protection

Although the sun produces vitamin D for our bodies, we need to be careful when it comes to sun exposure. Most of the wrinkles on your face and 90 percent of all skin cancers are probably due to sun damage, also referred to as photoaging. To minimize sun damage, try to avoid being in direct sunlight when the sun's rays are harshest—between 10 A.M. and 3 P.M.—and when you do go outdoors, regardless of the hour or the sun's intensity, always wear a sunscreen of SPF 15 or higher. It's best to apply your sunscreen at least 20 to 30 minutes before heading out and to reapply it a few times a day. For the most effective product, look on the ingredient label for Parsol (also known as avobenzone) to protect you from UVA rays, and natural minerals like titanium dioxide or zinc oxide to protect you from UVB rays. Z-cote, a microfine version of zinc oxide, is said to offer protection from both UVA and UVB rays.

Stop Smoking

Go see a therapist or hypnotist, get the patch—do whatever it takes to get off the cigarettes. Do this not only for your overall health but also because smoking is a major cause of massive skin damage (sun damage is the biggest one). Smoking is damaging in two ways. First, constant facial movements result in lines. Second, a buildup of tar narrows the blood vessels that in turn nourish the skin. The result is that the skin doesn't recover as well from injuries like sun damage.

Those Burning Rays

Exposure to ultraviolet rays (UVA and UVB) in sunlight causes a steep drop in protective antioxidants and stimulates a tremendous amount of free-radical formation that can damage the outside and inside of your body. UVB rays are what cause the outer layer of skin to burn; UVA rays inflict major damage to the underlying layers of skin—the dermis and the subcutaneous layer. Both rays combined cause your skin's elastic fibers and collagen to dramatically break down. This kind of damage shows up as parched, leathery, wrinkled skin and potentially as skin cancer and cataracts.

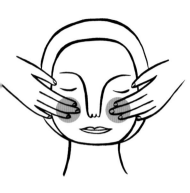

Bathe in Moisture

Water is the cheapest and most effective moisturizer, so drink up. When ingested, water oxygenates and optimizes metabolism through your entire body, most notably in the brain, liver, and kidneys. It also keeps your excretory functions working at their optimal best. Water is absolutely essential for proper hydration, keeping the skin moist, supple, soft, and clear. Get eight glasses of purified (bottled) or filtered (through a faucet attachment) water every day—and no, other liquids are *not* substitutes. If your water supply is chlorinated, put a filter on your showerhead so you don't absorb chloroform gas (trihalomethanes) into your lungs and skin.

Get Physical and Get Rest

Exercise benefits the skin by increasing blood circulation, which in turn provides nutrition to your skin cells and helps expel toxins, control stress, and promote deep, revitalizing sleep. And speaking of sleep, it may be your downtime, but it's when your skin—and, in fact, your entire body—is busy regenerating, renewing, and rebuilding tissue.

Choosing Skin-Care Products

What you put on your skin and how you put it on plays a significant role in your skin's long-term beauty. Products that contain inferior ingredients can ultimately harm skin by drying it out, clogging pores, irritating it, or causing allergic reactions. That's why organic is the only way to go. Organic skin-care products contain certified organic plant extracts and whole foods, which are by definition free of the damaging plastics and toxic substances used in many nonorganic skin-care products. If you must reach for a nonorganic product, make sure to read the ingredients label and avoid anything with petrochemicals, synthetic fragrances, artificial colors, preservatives, harsh detergents, and alcohol.

Beyond organic store-bought skin-care products, you can also make your own products—including some simple yet very effective cleansers, toners, and moisturizers. I can't stress the following enough, though: Never use out-of-date or rancid food products (yogurt and some oils have *definite* expiration dates); always be mindful of any ingredients that require the final concoction to be refrigerated; and be sure to thoroughly rinse off any skin-care product. Believe it or not, skin-care professionals often see clients with fungus or staph infections brought on by skin-care products containing spoiled ingredients.

Regardless of the products you choose, always use a gentle massaging movement when manipulating your skin. Rough tugging, rubbing, or abrasive handling with your fingers, towels, tissues, or machines can damage your skin. Look for 100 percent natural and organic cotton fiber tissues.

Vitamins for Your Skin

Many skin-care products today contain vitamins. When applied topically, these products are said to improve the skin's appearance. Time and further testing will tell if these claims are genuine, but for now there is some limited evidence of the following benefits.

Vitamin A assists in hydration. It is also a key element in some exfoliating procedures used to reduce fine lines and control acne.

Vitamin C aids in hydration and is also an antioxidant that's very healing for damaged underlying skin tissue. It enhances collagen production, firms and tightens skin, and reduces lines. It also improves blood supply to your skin, giving it a more youthful glow. Use caution with products containing vitamin C, however, as they can irritate sensitive, dry, and mature skin types.

Vitamin E is hydrating and an antioxidant. It is excellent for healing skin, fading scars, and reducing the appearance of stretch marks.

Vitamin D is essential for great skin and teeth.

Vitamin K can help fade broken capillaries, spider veins, and bruises. It also speeds healing of sun-damaged skin.

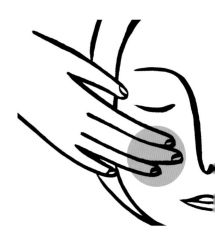

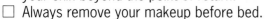

Here are some quick tips that will help you have healthy, radiant skin.

☐ Say so long to hot baths. Hot water zaps the moisture out of your skin. Your best bet? Take a warm shower instead.
☐ Don't sleep with your face scrunched into a pillow. Cumulatively, this can stretch your skin beyond the point of return.
☐ Always remove your makeup before bed.
☐ Smile! Your face tends to conform to the expressions you wear.

Your Skin-Care Regimen

When the foundation of good health has been laid by making the most of sunshine, fresh air, sleep, water, and food, it will be time to turn to the little details concerning the care of the complexion, hair, teeth, and nails.

A desirable skin-care regimen includes five steps: cleansing, toning, moisturizing, exfoliating, and protecting. Aside from exfoliating, which is generally done once a week, you can perform the other four steps every day or according to your individual skin-care needs. You may also choose to visit a schooled and certified skin-care professional for facial treatments. As a matter of fact, I recommend it, especially when the seasons change and your skin is probably changing, too. You can find reputable skin-care specialists through your dermatologist, at all spas, or possibly through your beauty salon.

As you continue reading about the five skin-care steps, please note that I've supplied common organic ingredients appropriate for each skin type. This is by no means a definitive list. Check "Recommended Reading and Resources" on page 134 and visit a reputable health food store for more suggestions.

Cleansing

Generally, you should cleanse your skin twice a day. For damaged or very dry skin, cleanse only once a day, in the evening or morning, and at the other time simply splash your face with filtered water and follow with a gentle toner and then a moisturizer. Use gentle movements for cleansing both facial and body skin. On your face and neck, use upward and outward strokes. Around your delicate upper eye area, work from the inner corner out. Around your bottom eye area, work from the outer corner in.

Many soap bars are alkaline, which can disturb your skin's natural acid mantle. Reach for glycerin or olive oil–based soaps—they're excellent for normal to oily skins. Look for all-natural, ph-balanced soaps. Cleansing lotions, creams, or milks, as well as oils (such as almond, avocado, borage, evening primrose, and hazelnut) are superb for removing makeup, dead surface cells, dirt, and grime from all skin types. They're especially good for dry skin because these treatments leave behind an emollient film that prevents excessive loss of natural oil. Some mornings I use sweet almond oil to massage my entire body (including my face) before stepping into the shower. The almond oil serves as my cleanser and moisturizer.

Study cleanser container labels before you buy, and choose products with ingredients that are best for your skin type.

Oily skin benefits from cleansers with aloe vera, camphor oils, chamomile, eucalyptus, menthol, or witch hazel.

Dry and sensitive skin calls for allantoin, aloe vera, coconut oil, hyaluronic acid, or kelp.

Aging skin reacts well to allantoin, kelp, olive oil, peppermint oil, shea butter, vegetable glycerin, and vitamins A, C, and E.

Toning

Toners, appropriate for every skin type, reduce the size of pores and remove cleanser residue. No alcohol, please! This or any similarly harsh toner removes too much oil, throws the skin off balance, and ultimately can increase oil production. What you want

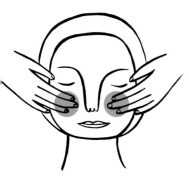

is a gentle toner within an acceptable acid range. For extra sensory pleasure, you may want to try toners containing herbs or essential oils, available at health food stores. To apply these toners, follow the manufacturer's directions printed on the label.

My favorite toner is rosewater, a centuries-old secret for glowing skin. Pure rose essential oil can be expensive—it takes 2,000 pounds of rose petals to extract 1 pound of essential oil—but it's worth it. Rosewater comes from this distillation process used to make rose essential oil. You can find rosewater at most Middle Eastern food stores; keep your rosewater refrigerated after purchasing. You can mist rosewater over cleansed skin or whisk a cotton pad dampened with rosewater over your skin in gentle upward, outward movements. You can do this over your face and body at intervals throughout the day.

There are wonderful organic toners out there for every skin type. Toners containing burdock or nettle are refreshing for all skin types. Toners containing apple cider vinegar, lavender, lemon, or sage and are all beneficial for oily skin. Calendula, made into a tea and cooled, is a wonderful toner for sensitive skin. Make small batches (about 8 ounces) and remix fresh toner every 1 to 2 weeks. Store this toner in the refrigerator. Apply with a damp cotton ball. Chamomile is calming and antiallergenic to inflamed, sensitive skin. If you like a witch hazel toner, try adding honey or vitamin E to balance the witch hazel's drying effect. And, of course, the best toner is cool water. Splash it on your face after cleansing to tighten and close the pores, and use a spray attachment in the shower to direct a cold spritz over your entire body.

Moisturizing

For maximum moisturizing power, look for lotions with natural emollients and humectants. Some of the very best include aloe vera, soy, vegetable glycerin, and vegetable or nut oils (like almond, avocado, olive, and sesame oils). Grapeseed and kukai are superb for oilier skins. Moisturizing essential fatty acids are

The Patch Test

There is always the possibility of an allergic reaction to any product or ingredient, whether synthesized in a laboratory or by nature, when applied to the skin. This includes essential oils. To avoid potential problems, mix a drop of essential oil with ½ teaspoon of plant oil. Rub a small amount of this mix into the fold of your elbow and wait 24 hours. If redness or irritation develops, choose an alternative product or essential oil and repeat the patch test.

found in evening primrose and borage oils, and in addition look for shea and cocoa butters, rose water, honey, and iris. Alpha hydroxy acids (AHAs) in moisturizing lotions make marvelous emollients, due to their gentle exfoliation abilities and natural protection against moisture loss. If you choose to use a moisturizer with AHAs, follow the instructions carefully and consider skipping AHA exfoliants as a separate process. You don't want to overdo.

Humectants provide a layer of protection to the skin barrier, drawing moisture to the skin and preventing internal moisture levels from evaporating. Glycerin is a popular and effective humectant, and you should use a form that is naturally derived.

On a deeper level, moisturizers can also condition, repair, and protect. For mature or aging skin, look for products containing essential fatty acids, liposomes, or hyaluronic acid. Moisturizers with liposomes deliver nourishment to your skin's dermal layer, increasing your skin's internal water-binding capacity. Aloe vera is a great moisturizer for all skin types, and when aloe vera juice is applied with a damp cotton pad, it becomes a toner and moisturizer.

To receive maximum benefits from your moisturizer, try these easy suggestions.

- Apply moisturizers to slightly damp skin and lock in valuable extra moisture.

- Don't over-moisturize with gloppy, heavy, or greasy creams. Your skin needs to breathe!

- Give your eye area extra attention and moisturizer, since this skin tends to age earliest. And please, be as gentle as possible!

- Lightly pat moisturizer around your eye area with the pad of your middle or ring finger. Don't tug at your skin!

- Don't forget to moisturize your neck, a graceful extension of your face.

All about AHAs

Also called fruit acids, AHAs encourage the top layer of dead skin cells to slough off. New skin cells are generated and the skin's surface is refreshed. Benefits may include a reduced appearance of fine lines and wrinkles, a lightening of age spots, and fewer blemishes. Some examples include glycolic acid from sugar cane, lactic acid from milk, tannic acid from grapes, malic acid from apples, citric acid from citrus fruits, and mandelic acid from bitter almonds. AHAs can make the skin exceptionally sensitive to UV rays, so sunscreen becomes even more important. If you see prolonged irritation or reddening of your skin, discontinue use.

Exfoliating

Exfoliating your skin is integral to removing the top dead layers of skin cells and debris, encouraging better cell turnover, and preventing clogged pores. Depending on your skin type, exfoliation may need to be done more or less often, but minimally once a week. Chemical peels provide maximum exfoliation, although these should be done no more than once a year and only by a skin-care professional. AHAs may be used at home, but then it's up to you to monitor product strengths and results. Home AHA products should have an acid concentration no higher than 10 percent. An acid concentration above 10 percent should only be administered by a dermatologist. The pH should not be less than 3.5 or higher than 4. If your product is too strong, you strip away too much of your skin's natural acid mantle and consequently throw your skin into imbalance. Skin-care professionals recommend applying AHAs according to the product label instructions—just once a week if you have dry skin, and up to two times a week if you have oilier skin.

Special Treatments

Here are a few luxurious techniques for treating your skin. These may be incorporated into your five skin-care steps or used independently for extra nourishing care of your skin.

Natural Masks and Exfoliants

Masks deep-cleanse the pores and reduce pore size. Some masks serve double-duty as exfoliants. They are applied and left on for up to 20 minutes, as opposed to an exfoliant, which is generally applied and then immediately rinsed. Carefully follow the directions for your individual skin-care product.

To slough off dead surface cells, you can purchase products that contain alpha hydroxy acids (AHAs) or are granular in nature, or you can make your own. The enzymes in banana, cream, honey, lemon, oatmeal, papaya, pineapple, salt, strawberry, and sugar are but a few natural ways to deep cleanse and nourish the skin. You can also strengthen the toning, tightening, or hydrating effect of store-bought products by adding one or more of these ingredients. Here are a few of the many possibilities.

● Mix 2 tablespoons of ground oatmeal with ½ tablespoon of almond oil and ½ tablespoon of honey. Stroke over your face and neck, and gently massage in. Leave on for up to 20 minutes. Rinse thoroughly, then apply moisturizer. This mix is very hydrating, deep cleansing, and balancing for all skin types. (This recipe works wonderfully on your entire body. The quantities here make enough for only your face, so adjust your quantities for full-body application.)

● Mash fruit and place it directly on your skin. Use banana or avocado pulp for dry skin, banana or pineapple for sensitive skin, and strawberry or green papaya for oily skin. For dry skin, add a small amount of honey to accentuate the moisturizing effect. Apply after cleansing. Leave on for up to 20 minutes.

● Mash a cucumber into a fine pulp and mix with enough organic powdered milk to make an easily spreadable cream. This makes a marvelous hydrating and drawing mask, pulling impurities and excess oil from pores.

● Make a natural, gently abrasive facial scrub by mixing 1 tablespoon of baking soda with enough almond oil to create a moderately thick cream. Massage delicately into facial skin. Rinse well, pat dry, and then apply moisturizer.

A Word of Caution

If you want to work with essential oils, it's a good idea to consult with a health-care practitioner or a qualified aromatherapist first. Essential oils are concentrated and volatile, and therefore can be harmful if used improperly. Never ingest essential oils. Most essential oils should be diluted in a plant oil before being applied to the skin or added to bath water, although you would use undiluted oils in diffusers. Some essential oils should not be used during pregnancy or when certain health problems exist, such as low or high blood pressure. Check with your doctor if you have any of these conditions. And always keep essential oils away from your eyes and away from children.

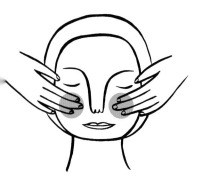

● Make a salt scrub for your body skin by mixing ½ cup of fine sea salt with 2 tablespoons of baking soda and ¼ cup of almond or olive oil. Gently massage over your entire body. Two to four drops of essential oils—lavender or ylang-ylang—help hydrate your skin.

● Create a mask of cornmeal and clay, both excellent ingredients to gently balance oilier skins. Or, look for these ingredients in store-bought organic skin-care products. You have a wide variety of clays to choose from, including green, red, black, yellow, Fuller's Earth, and kaolin clay. Mix with a small amount of water until it's the consistency of paste. You may also add a small amount of yogurt or honey (still aiming for a pastelike consistency) for their moisturizing benefits.

Massage

I am an avid believer in the power of massage. When you combine massage therapy with yoga, tai chi, chiropractic, or acupuncture, you experience healthful results in all your bodily functions. There are a wide variety of massage therapies to choose from, including Ayurvedic, Swedish, shiatsu, accupressure reflexology, and cranial sacral therapy. No matter what type of massage you prefer, know that your skin, as well as your entire mind-body physiology, will profoundly respond to and benefit from it.

Whether you visit a professional massage therapist, enjoy a massage by the hands of a loved one, or treat yourself to a self-massage, you'll feel cared for, loved, and touched on a sensory level that is incredibly blissful. It's been shown that the power of touch may reduce stress, increase levels of endorphins (natural pain suppressers), ease back pain, fight anorexia and bulimia, lift depression, and lower blood pressure. In addition to all these benefits, massage can also increase the flow of blood and lymph throughout the system, making this a primary method for detoxification. Tiffany M. Field, Ph.D., founder and director of The Touch Research Institute at The University of Miami School of Medicine, believes massage can even impact the bottom line where you work. She cites a study where workers given 15-minute massages twice a week for 5 weeks performed better on the job than did those who did not receive rubdowns. (For more information on massage, see "Recommended Reading and Resources" on page 134.)

Here's the Rub

I think you will find the following self-massage technique incredibly healing and detoxifying. Enjoy it in the morning, coupled with meditation and yoga, to help put everything into glorious perspective. As you try the following technique, adjust the amount of pressure you apply to your body. Some people prefer a light touch, some prefer firm pressure, and still others want a more vigorous massage for its stimulating qualities. Do what feels most natural and pleasant to you.

This daily self-massage is best done in the morning before bathing or showering. Choose organic plant oils labeled "pure cold" or "expeller pressed" as your base massage oil. This ensures that chemical pesticide and fertilizer residues will not be applied to and absorbed through your skin. Sesame oil is a good all-around selection because of its ability to be absorbed and for its potent antioxidant qualities. For dry skin, you might want to use oils like almond and avocado, or ghee (clarified butter) instead. For oily skin, you might choose almond, canola, grapeseed, kukui, mustard, or safflower oils. Use a minimal amount on oilier skin. For sensitive skins, use cooling oils like almond, coconut, olive, or sunflower oils. Any of these oils are balancing for normal skin. Do not use mineral oil, as it can be quite drying and will not penetrate your skin.

Scented Massage Oil

Massage will delight your sense of smell as well as touch when you add aromatic essential oils to your massage oil. To make a mixed oil, combine 1 ounce of your base oil with 15 drops of any essential oil in a small bottle with a dispenser top. For more details about essential oils and their properties and sensory effects, please refer to "Organic Beauty for the Senses" on page 91. Depending on your personal preference, you can blend different oils in desired proportions. If you like, you can warm this oil mix to body temperature before applying it by placing the dispenser bottle in a bowl of very hot water for a few minutes.

Water is the most healing of all remedies, and

Here's the Ayurvedic self-massage approach, called Abhyanga, that I teach in the "Creating Health" courses offered through Infinite Possibilities Knowledge, the educational arm of Deepak Chopra's company.

1. *Stand or sit on a large bath towel*. The towel catches any oil drips.
2. *Begin massaging your head first*. Take about a minute for this. Pour a small amount of oil into your palms and work it evenly onto the fingertips and palms. Begin at the top front of your forehead and using the pads of your fingertips, massage in small circular motions. Work back to the crown area. Move your entire scalp to render it more flexible. Work from the temple areas back to the lower crown area. Lastly, work in small circular strokes from behind your ears to the center nape. Use more oil as needed.
3. *Next, move to your face*. With a small amount of oil, work gently over your face using outward and upward movements. Gently work around your eye area—outward along the top brow area, and inward along the underneath area. Use a light patting motion under your eyes. Gently massage and knead around the outer ear lobe area and stroke behind your ears. Stroke the front of your neck with upward motions and the back of your neck with up and down strokes.
4. *Stroke back and forth over the area between your neck and shoulders, using circular clockwise motions over your shoulders*. With your palm and fingers, stroke back and forth over the top of your arm and forearm, switching to circular strokes over your elbows and wrists. Massage each finger, stroking upward on the back of your hand toward the wrist. Massage in a circular clockwise fashion in the center palm area.
5. *Over your chest, heart, and abdomen*, use gentle, circular clockwise strokes.
6. *Reaching behind to your lower back and buttocks, massage in a circular motion*. Going as far up as possible, stroke back and forth on your upper back.
7. *Now move to your legs*. Use long back and forth strokes on your upper leg (front and back), smaller circular strokes at your knee, and long back and forth strokes on your lower leg (front and back). Continue down to your ankles.

the best of all cosmetics.
Old Arabian proverb

8. Use upward strokes along the tops of your feet. Then gently massage each toe. Briskly stroke back and forth along your soles.

Allow your attention to be fully present and on your body. Breathe smoothly, deeply, and evenly as you massage. Try not to have any distractions. This entire process will allow your mind to profoundly settle down.

If possible, relax for 5 to 10 minutes after your massage and before bathing. Use a gentle cleanser and tepid water to shower or bathe.

If you find that time prohibits a full-body self-massage, then concentrate on the scalp and feet. These are both rich energy centers for inducing a deep sense of relaxation. I particularly enjoy massaging my feet with oil and then covering them with organic cotton socks before bed. I also recommend a soothing massage of the abdomen, which helps digestion and tones this area.

This self-pampering ritual is one that will benefit anyone. It has a very stabilizing and grounding effect, while also enhancing alertness and preparing you to better face each day.

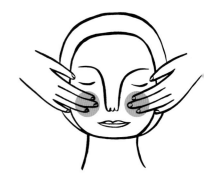

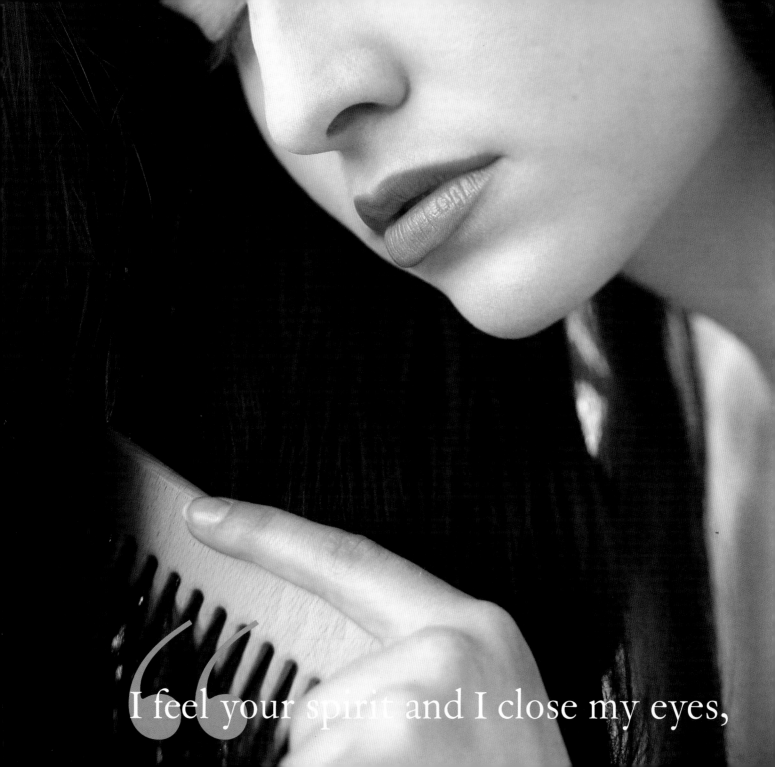

"I feel your spirit and I close my eyes,

the language of *hair*

Knowing the bright hair blowing in the sun.

Sara Teasdale

Since the beginning of time, powerful **symbolism** has been braided into the idea of hair. Early caveman hauled his woman away by her hair. Medieval knights rode off into battle wearing a snip of their lady's pubic hair tucked inside a locket. In Native American tradition, a lock of **hair** represented good medicine that would bring luck, health, and happiness. And the good or bad fortunes of Samson and Delilah, Rapunzel, and Lady Godiva all revolved around hair. ● Beyond fairy tales and **folklore**, hair dramatically influences how we feel about our total image. When Yale University conducted a study on the psychological effects of a bad hair day, they found that people's self-esteem goes awry when their hair goes askew. **Men and women** suffering from unmanageable hair tend to feel less smart, less sociable, and less capable. ● Considering the significance we give hair, it's no surprise that worldwide we spend billions of dollars on hair products and services. We cut, color, curl, straighten, comb, and brush. We buy hair products to cleanse, condition, smooth, **shine**, detangle, and hold. We expect our hair to express our identity, our **moods**, and our desires. We have created an entire language spoken through hair.

The Nature of Hair

You have over 5 million hair follicles on your body. The only place where you won't find hair is on your lips, the palms of your hands, and the soles of your feet. Each hair springs from a follicle in your skin's dermal layer, and each hair has its own blood, nerve, and muscle supply. At the base of the hair follicle, the papilla, or hair root, is fed a rich supply of oxygenated blood via the capillaries. This is vital for healthy hair growth. If your mind-body physiology experiences imbalances or toxicity, you can be fairly certain you'll see the effects in the condition of your hair. Stress, environmental toxins, poor diet, hormonal fluctuations, illness, the use of pharmaceutical or illicit drugs—they all play an integral role in nourishing or not nourishing your hair.

Am I Losing My Hair?

We all lose from 50 to 100 hairs each day. If you experience hair loss outside this range, you need to determine whether this is due to a medical condition requiring a physician's attention or due to a temporary condition. Temporary hair loss may occur because you recently suffered a trauma, extreme stress, a dramatic change in diet, or something equally disruptive to your mind-body physiology. Hormonal disruptions or changes, whether induced by lifestyle choices, heredity, or the natural aging process, are the primary causes of hair loss. A physician should check your hormone levels and prescribe an appropriate course of action if hormones are to blame.

The hair we see is keratin, a hard protein made of 97 percent protein and 3 percent moisture. This explains why it is absolutely vital that you get an ample supply of protein and water from your daily diet. It also illustrates the importance of using external products that introduce protein to strengthen and fortify your hair. Furthermore, to maintain your hair's natural shine, pliability, and resiliency, you want to be sure and get rich moisturizing elements into it.

Your hair's strength, resiliency, and moisture content are defined by its elasticity and porosity—two separate yet interconnected qualities. In a healthy state, hair is resilient, has good elasticity, and bounces back. Hair that is compromised in any way may lose its elasticity, and protein-rich hair-care products may be needed to build up, strengthen, and help hair achieve its optimal condition. Moisture-starved hair is generally porous, resulting in hair that feels brittle and breaks easily. Treatments that replenish moisture *and* protein equalize your hair's porosity and simultaneously enhance elasticity.

Organically Beautiful Hair—From Within

The factors that affect your hair growth (as well as loss) include your general state of health, age, environment, inherited genes, and lifestyle—specifically your nutritional intake, physical activity level, and ability to handle life stress. Each of these factors plays a direct role in either nurturing or damaging your hair and scalp.

Nutrition for Your Scalp and Hair

As with your skin, eating a balanced, whole-foods, organic diet that's rich in vegetables, fruits, lean proteins, complex carbohydrates, and monounsaturated fats will ultimately give you strong, resilient, shiny hair. Foods rich in silicon will strengthen hair. This includes green and red peppers, potato skins, and sprouts. Sea vegetables, including kelp, are also good for your hair. And do consider a high-quality multivitamin and mineral complex.

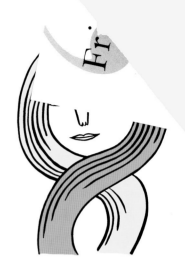

Make sure your diet includes the recommended daily allowance of essential fatty acids. This will keep you well lubricated inside and out. If your hair doesn't seem to be growing very fast, or if it's thinning out, a deficiency in essential fatty acids may be the culprit. Dr. Andrew Weil, director of the program in integrative medicine at the University of Arizona, recommends taking GLA (gamma linolenic acid) supplements in the form of black currant, borage, or evening primrose oils. Take 500 milligrams twice a day. After 6 to 8 weeks, you should begin to see results, including healthier hair and healthier skin! Dr. Weil also recommends increasing your consumption of omega-3 fatty acids by eating more salmon, mackerel, and herring, or by taking a supplement of flax seeds (1 to 2 tablespoons a day, ground and then sprinkled over food) or flaxseed oil (1 tablespoon a day).

Naturally, get those eight glasses of purified water every day! Your hair's resiliency and shine depends on it. Please try to limit your intake of coffee, refined carbohydrates, saturated fats, salt, and sugar. These, along with denatured food consumption, inactivity, and stress, can truly alter your hair's health. (Denatured

How Many Hairs?

We each have anywhere from 90,000 to 140,000 hairs on our head, and while I'm not so sure blondes have more fun, I am certain they have more hair. Blondes generally have 140,000 hairs, brunettes have around 110,000, black hair comes in around 108,000, and redheads have around 90,000.

foods include all edibles devoid of the life force—the energy and intelligence—that makes for the finest mind-body physiology, and include foods that have pesticide residues; chemical, antibiotic, and hormone additives; artificial flavorings; and so on.)

Scalp Health

The health of your scalp is intimately related to the health of your hair. A hard, thickened, or tight scalp, as well as a pimply, itchy, scaly, oily, or dry scalp, may indicate internal health problems as well as improper scalp care. These conditions almost always affect your hair. By using gentle cleansers and conditioners, rinsing thoroughly, and giving your scalp a daily massage, you can alleviate some of these adverse conditions.

Another biggie when it comes to impacting scalp health is stress. Reduce it! Giving in to stress can worsen dandruff as well as other skin conditions. Exercise, meditate, do your deep breathing, yoga, or tai chi—whatever it takes to bring perspective and calm into your life.

Dandruff Woes

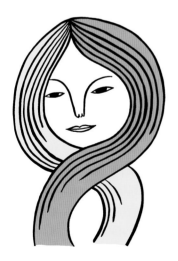

While there are medical causes for dandruff, a dry, flaky scalp is sometimes misdiagnosed and is not dandruff at all. Sometimes what appears to be dandruff is actually flaking caused by an intense buildup of hair-care products on the scalp, or insufficient massaging of the scalp to slough off cellular tissue. If, despite better rinsing and more massage, you're still plagued by persistent dandruff, psoriasis, or contact or seborrheic dermatitis, then see your hair-care professional, primary care physician, or dermatologist for the proper treatments.

I do want to offer one word of caution when it comes to over-the-counter as well as prescription dandruff shampoos: These products can be harsh and should be used for the briefest amount of time needed to be effective. As soon as possible, return to a gentle, organically oriented approach. You can find wonderful treatments for dandruff

snapdragons pleading for water.
Paul Gardner

that are quite natural and organic at your health food store. Shampoos with zinc oxide offer a more natural way to go, rather than dandruff shampoos containing coal tar, a petroleum derivative and a known carcinogen. Zinc oxide in shampoo also serves as a hair sunscreen and conditioner.

Here are a few more suggestions to better control or alleviate dandruff. Again, if after a week the problem persists, you should check in with a hair-care professional, physician, or dermatologist.

● Consider adding 3 to 5 drops of tea tree oil—the wonder antiseptic— to a dime- or quarter-size amount (depending on hair length) of gentle shampoo. Or, look for shampoos and conditioners that contain tea tree oil.

● Gently massage organic olive oil into the scalp (leave it on overnight, if possible), followed by a gentle brushing with a soft-bristle brush and cleansing with a gentle shampoo.

● Ginger, a tremendous anti-inflammatory agent, is another aid for controlling dandruff. Mix one part purified water to one part ginger tea, and rinse your hair with this combination. You can also add equal amounts of plant oil, such as jojoba, olive, sesame, or sweet almond oil, to the juice from freshly grated ginger, and massage the mixture into your scalp before bed. Rinse it out in the morning.

Scalp and Hair Treatments
Using a natural or organic hair rinse can be a delightful experience, as well as a great way to remedy a variety of discomforts and problems. Here are a few simple ideas for make-it-yourself hair rinses. Unless otherwise indicated, you make herbal tea rinses by

steeping about 2 tablespoons of dried herbs in 1 cup of boiling water. Let the mixture cool, then strain the herbs off before using. Adjust formula amounts according to your own hair's length and needs. You can also add 3 to 5 drops of essential oils for their aromatic as well as therapeutic properties.

● To combat an itchy, dry scalp, use one of my favorite hair rinses after shampooing and conditioning. Make a strong organic herbal tea with 1 to 2 tablespoons each of comfrey, nettles, and rosemary (witch hazel and thyme may also be added or substituted) in 2 cups of water.

● An herbal tea rinse made with chamomile adds gloss and highlights to lighter hair. A tea made from the root of oriental (panax) ginseng replenishes moisture, giving the hair more flexibility and sheen.

● Try a lavender rinse to restore hair's silkiness and shine, or try a lemongrass rinse to condition hair, making it soft and lustrous.

● A rinse with yarrow tea improves hair's manageability.

● To balance and condition oilier hair and scalps, use either a rinse of 2 tablespoons of apple cider vinegar mixed with 1 cup of water or an herbal tea rinse of 1 tablespoon of rosemary and 1 tablespoon of sage. This second rinse has a few additional benefits. The rosemary acts as a great detangler and adds shine to darker hair. The sage can cumulatively be used to cover those occasional gray hairs in medium to dark brown and black hair.

"The roots of a plant go down, and the deeper

Magic in the Bottle

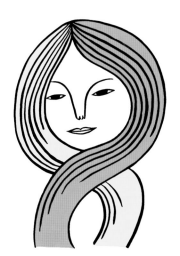

Some of the most important hair-care choices you'll make are your shampoo and conditioner. Read the labels on mass-marketed shampoo bottles, and it truly sounds like they perform magic. You see words like luxurious, full, beautiful—but the promises are often stronger than the results. Instead, I suggest you find an organic shampoo and conditioner. There are plenty of good choices on the market. Shampoos and conditioners with organic plant extracts, essential oils, and whole-food derivatives do for the hair and scalp what they do for the body, providing a high level of vitamins, minerals and trace minerals, enzymes, amino acids, essential fatty acids, phytosterols, and natural sugars. They strengthen, hydrate, relax, stimulate, and detoxify your hair and scalp, and the results can indeed feel and look like real magic.

When it comes to a shampoo, you want a gentle, organic cleanser. This protects your hair's natural oils from being stripped and consequently safeguards your hair and scalp's natural acid pH of 4.5 to 5.5—a neutral or balanced pH is 7.0. Anything above this is alkaline. Just as something that is too acid can be detrimental to your hair, so can anything that is too alkaline. To protect your hair, be sure to read labels, and look for shampoos that contain natural purifying and cleansing herbs (like basil, biloba, comfrey, ginko, and yarrow to name but a few), along with essential oils.

It is desirable that shampoos and conditioners, be both humectant and emollient. These qualities describe a product's ability to draw and hold moisture into the hair from the environment, as well as its ability to prevent further loss of moisture from the hair. For optimum moisturizing power, look for one or more of the following natural ingredients on your shampoo and conditioner label: aloe, avocado, banana, burdock, calendula, carrot puree, chamomile, comfrey, cucumber, glycerin, honey, kelp, lecithin, marshmallow, milk, molasses, nettle, pear or apple juice, plant oils, and shea butter. Many of these ingredients provide a few extra benefits, as well. Some offer a measure of protein, as do wheat, soy, rice, milk, oats, alfalfa, and black beans. Since hair is predominantly made of protein, applying protein-rich products directly onto your hair may

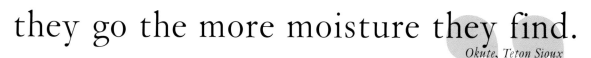

they go the more moisture they find.

Okute, Teton Sioux

Hair style is the final tip-off whether or not a

act to shore up weaknesses within each hair strand and optimize your hair's elasticity and porosity. Some ingredients, such as yarrow and burdock, offer natural astringency. Then there are citrus fruit oils (grapefruit, lemon, lime, and orange), apple cider vinegar, eucalyptus, peppermint, sage, and rosemary, which all act to smooth the cuticle and create incredible shine. Rosemary and peppermint are effective for stimulating hair growth, as are spearmint and all the citrus fruits.

Stimulating Hair Growth

Aromatherapy is being touted as a possible solution for hair loss or thinning. In a study published in *Archives of Dermatology*, Scottish researchers showed that a daily massage using certain essential oils mixed into a carrier plant oil was three times more effective at stimulating hair growth than a massage with the use of a carrier oil alone.

To try the treatment used in this study, mix 2 drops each of thyme and cedarwood essential oils, 3 drops each of lavender and rosemary essential oils, and ¾ ounce of grapeseed oil. Massage into the scalp for a few minutes, then wrap a shower cap or a warm towel around the head for 30 minutes. Finally, rinse out with a gentle shampoo. This is also a wonderful moisturizing treatment.

This treatment is quite safe, however if you are pregnant or have high blood pressure, diabetes, or epilepsy, check with your doctor before using this aromatherapy treatment.

Preserve and Protect

It is important that the products we use have a natural preservative in them to retard spoilage, inhibit the formation of bacteria, and provide protection from harmful oxidizing agents. Natural preservatives include citric acid; grapefruit seed extract; vitamins A, C, and E; and wheat germ. Look for these ingredients on hair-care product labels. When natural preservatives are used, either in part or entirely, the need for traditional, synthesized chemical preservatives is reduced.

You also want hair formulas to contain antiseptics—ingredients that destroy or inhibit the growth of problematic scalp organisms even after you've rinsed out the hair formula. Many herbs serve beautifully as natural antiseptics. Such herbs include but are not limited to aloe, burdock, chamomile, rosemary, sage, and the wonderfully versatile tea tree oil.

Strengthen Your Hair Treatments

Whether it's a shampoo, conditioner, or massage oil, you can pump up store-bought products by mixing organic ingredients either into the product bottle or into the portion of the product you are using

woman really knows herself.

Hubert de Givenchy

at that moment. For instance, add a few drops of rosemary essential oil to your shampoo or your massage oil. Or add an organic egg—with its high protein levels—to your shampoo or conditioner. Use aloe vera, honey, and plant oils as desired. Be creative, but also be careful. If you add an organic ingredient that can spoil, such as eggs or some oils, be sure to either keep the mixture refrigerated or remain mindful of its expiration date.

Don't limit yourself to the few hair-care recipes provided in this chapter—there are many wonderful books on the subject that will get you hooked on mixing your own hair tonics at home. I offer several excellent options in "Recommended Reading and Resources" on page 134.

Shampooing

We Americans shampoo the heck out of our hair! In many other countries, they shampoo less often and consequently enjoy healthier hair. I have to admit, however, that if I've been out in the elements and pollution, or if I've exercised, I do feel it is more healthful to shampoo every day—but I do so with a gentle, organic cleanser. Plus, hair does tend to look its most beautiful after being renewed with a good shampoo. The only exception to this would be fragile or very dry, overly porous hair. Shampooing every day may exacerbate these conditions. I think you get the idea—you need to be aware of what your hair needs on individual days, and shampoo accordingly.

In Top Condition

When it comes to shampoo's partner—the conditioner—the number-one comment I hear is that conditioner can weigh hair down, particularly fine hair. However, if the conditioner has been elegantly formulated and if it does not contain heavy waxes or polymers, this should not be a concern.

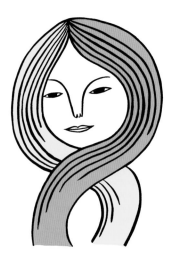

Conditioner categories include daily rinse-out, leave-in, and deep-penetrating.

Daily rinse-outs are generally used in the shower to detangle, even out porosity, prevent moisture loss, and (to some degree) provide thermal and UV protection.

A leave-in conditioner is applied and left in, serving to protect the hair from styling and heat exposure—sun included. I equate this to a moisturizer smoothed on the skin before applying foundation. A leave-in conditioner also assists in smoothing the cuticle, reduces friction while styling, calms static, and controls frizziness.

Deep-penetrating moisturizing and protein treatments help revitalize hair that's been damaged from chemical services, harsh hair products, damage from brushing or styling, or damage from fun in the sun and water. Speaking of outdoor activities, you should rinse, shampoo, and deep condition after every plunge into sea or pool water. Some people even slather on a deep protein conditioner before going outdoors to play and rinse it off after returning inside. Of course, one of the simplest ways to safeguard your hair is with a hat. Any hat helps, but you might want to look for a hat that actually offers extra protection against ultraviolet rays (the hat label should loudly proclaim this attribute). These hats are available at many department and specialty stores.

Conditioners You Can Make

Whether you shop online, at a health food store, or at a salon or spa, there are many magnificent organic conditioners available. There are also many opportunities for dabbling in your 100 percent organic kitchen!

For dry hair, make a smoothie conditioner with a small, ripe banana mixed with a bit of honey and sweet almond oil. Work the mixture into your hair and scalp after shampooing, cover your head with a shower cap, let everything sit for up to 30 minutes, and then rinse. Apple cider vinegar is a great at-home conditioner. It makes a great final rinse for oilier scalps and hair. Or, for normal hair, mix a couple tablespoons of aloe vera gel with a tablespoon of lemon juice for an after-shampoo rinse.

Another great once-a-week preshampoo treatment for damaged or very dry hair is a blend of avocado with jojoba oil. Gently work through the hair and scalp, wait 30 minutes, and then jump in the shower. Penetrating natural conditioners like aloe and plant oils are great for generally dry, curly hair. You can't go wrong with these delightful, tasty, aromatic ingredients. They're all chock full of good things like vitamins, minerals, essential fatty acids, and amino acids.

An Organic Hair-Care Routine

Now that you're savvy about how to choose a quality organic shampoo and conditioner, let's talk about how to use these products. Does it make a difference how you shampoo and condition your hair? Indeed it does. For the cleanest, most restorative results, follow this routine for beautiful hair. Some of the steps should be followed every time you shampoo, other steps—specifically some conditioning steps—can be used as often as you feel you hair needs them.

1. _Detangle your hair_ before shampooing. Use a natural bristle brush or your fingers to work through your hair.

2. _The best time to do a plant oil scalp and hair massage_ is right before stepping in the shower. Once in the shower, wet your hair down thoroughly.

3. _Work a small amount of shampoo_ between the palms of your hands and dab it onto your hair in several places. Don't worry about working lather through to the ends of your hair. Concentrate on massaging the scalp for at least 1 minute—3 is even better! Place the pads of your fingertips on your scalp and work from the front forehead toward the crown, then from the sides toward the center back, and lastly to the area behind the ears and on the nape of the neck. Use gentle back-and-forth and small circular motions. In this way, you cleanse your scalp and hair while also stimulating the blood flow to the scalp. Luxuriate in this step and do it mindfully. At intervals, draw your hands down through the length of your hair in one direction. Continue to gently massage your scalp, and never vigorously scrub or pile your hair. Keep in mind that organic and natural shampoos produce fewer suds, given their high level of certified organic plant extracts. Don't worry! Your hair is getting clean.

The Natural Look

Natural, shiny hair is organically beautiful hair. I think natural hair can be remarkably sexy—with a soft, approachable, tousled, moveable, and lived-in look. And by natural I don't mean letting your mane grow wild. Get a trim at least every 2 months. This keeps your shape fresh and prevents split ends. Remember, there is no product in the world capable of repairing split ends—despite what the label says!

Big Hair, Naturally

I've been called the Nettle Queen because of the nettle patch in my backyard garden and the many ways I use this wonderful herb. Taken internally, a nettles tea or tincture acts to purify the blood and serves as a wonderful tonic for the entire body. You can also apply the remarkably resinous herb externally to the hair by using a brewed nettles tea or by mixing a nettles tincture with water or your shampoo. To make a nettles tea rinse, which creates very full, voluminous hair, simmer a few tablespoons of dry nettle leaves in 2 cups of water for 30 minutes. Cool, strain, then pour this rinse over your hair after shampooing. Don't rinse it out. When mixing a nettles tincture with your shampoo, add several drops to a dollop of shampoo, and shampoo per the directions. Working with the nettles tincture stimulates blood circulation to your scalp, which in turn feeds your hair and ultimately optimizes healthy conditions for better hair growth.

4. *Rinse thoroughly with tepid water.* Hot water is drying and opens the cuticle. Hopefully you have nonchlorinated, soft water. (If not, consider buying a shower filter.) Rinse, rinse, and rinse some more, until you're absolutely positive all residue is gone from your hair and scalp. Rotate your body in a full circle under the showerhead and make sure that you let the water reach everywhere—especially underneath the layers of hair. Lift your hair out and away from your head as you continue to let water flow over it. Remember, many people who think they have dandruff are actually suffering from insufficient rinsing!

5. *Apply a rinse-out conditioner* and work it through with your fingers. Don't concentrate conditioners meant for the hair on the scalp area, and vice versa. After a minute, rinse thoroughly with tepid water.

6. *If you're using a deep protein or moisturizing treatment*, apply and leave it on for 5 to 10 minutes, then rinse. Taking this a step further, you could also finish shampooing and showering, step out of the shower, towel blot your hair, and then apply your treatment. Work it through your hair and place a plastic bag or shower cap over your hair. Your natural body heat will intensify the conditioning effect. Wait for 30 minutes, then rinse.

7. *After rinsing the conditioning treatment* out of your hair, regardless of which treatment you use, you could apply an apple cider or herbal vinegar rinse. This enhances your hair's shine, removes all residues from your hair and scalp, and in some cases treats scalp conditions such as dandruff. Apply the rinse in the shower with either a spray bottle or a color tint bottle. Saturate the lengths, leave on for a minute, then rinse.

8. *Gently squeeze,* pat, and towel-blot your hair with a thick organic cotton towel. This is essential to healthy hair. Don't aggressively rub, twist, or wring your hair with a towel or your hands. The friction can erode your hair's outer cuticle layer.

9. *Use a large-tooth comb* or your fingers to gently comb through a small amount of leave-in conditioner. Do not use a pick, fine-tooth comb, or bristle brush on wet hair! This will cause breakage and split ends. If your hair is long, begin the comb-out on the underneath layers, taking short strokes first at the ends, then from the middle to the ends, and finally from the scalp to the ends.

Color and Texture Services

A huge scope of color and texture services is available for hair. Both these services have great power to psychologically impact how we see ourselves. Color can cover gray, create a tonal change, introduce highlights, or dramatically alter your hair color. Texture services, such as a chemical relaxer or body wave, can add allover body and fullness, change directional patterns, or add volume and lift in only spot areas. Retexturizers chemically soften, manage, and relax highly curly textures. If you're wondering whether to try one of these treatments on your hair, here are some important factors to weigh before making a decision.

It's about Chemicals

Coloring, waving, and relaxing are all processes that require chemicals to change your hair's natural structure. Permanent hair colors change the natural pigment found within your hair. Demi-permanent color enriches color, adds shine, and blends gray. With its lower levels of hydrogen peroxide and artificial color molecules, this service has less structural impact on your hair then permanent color, and it gradually fades over a period of 4 to 6 weeks. Semi-permanent color stains your hair shaft and covers gray but fades after six to eight shampoos. Consider a natural color service or one that uses lower levels of hydrogen peroxide or developers, along with colors that have a lower dye lot. Whenever possible, choose temporary, semi-permanent, demi-permanent, and natural dyes over stronger, harsher permanent dyes, double processes, and progressive dyes.

Chemical waves and relaxers break and then re-form bonds within your hair. Sounds dramatic—and damaging. But rest assured, an experienced beauty professional can get the job done right. It's important to realize, however, that you are chemically changing your hair's natural structure. Diligent ongoing maintenance will be imperative to keep your hair looking good long after

Let Your Long Hair Be

If you have long hair, don't abuse it by subjecting it to long blow-drying sessions or repeated assaults with a curling iron. Instead, try drying your hair by loosely twisting and securing it at the top of your head. Or, you can loosely braid your hair. It's all about creating tousled organic texture without a lot of fuss or heat. Loose braiding and twisting are good techniques to use before you head out the door for work. After reaching the office, release your hair, toss your head forward, and finger comb.

your chemical treatment. Look for shampoos, conditioners, and styling products—preferably organic—appropriate for your specific chemical service.

Opt for waving or relaxing services that use the gentlest formula, and ask to have ammonium thioglycolate–free perms.

If you decide to try chemical services, space out the treatments so that there's time in between them to recondition and nurture your hair.

Natural and Herbal Color Rinses

Certified organic henna and plant materials can also color your hair, but with a more gentle and natural approach, since they contain no synthetic chemicals, preservatives, or harsh oxidizing chemicals, such as ammonia. These pure vegetable products do not alter the structure or natural color of your hair and actually condition your hair while imparting color and sheen. No matter what you have heard, these products have come a long way.

You can also create a wide variety of plant pigment color rinses yourself. These concoctions do not create a radical hair color change, but instead accentuate your hair's natural tone and shine. If your hair is less than 15 percent gray, some plants will disguise the gray. In these cases, the product actually stains your hair—although very subtly. Cumulative usage creates longer-lasting, slightly more intense results. You can repeat the application as often as desired, depending on the color level you prefer.

To make an herbal color rinse, add 2 to 4 tablespoons (depending on how intense you want the color) of your desired dried herb to 2 cups of filtered water. Using a nonaluminum pan, bring the mix to a boil, then simmer until the tea is reduced by about half. Let cool. I recommend straining this tea into a spray bottle.

Before you apply a color rinse, place a dark towel around your neck to catch drips. Thoroughly saturate your towel-dried hair with the solution. Do not rinse out. Dry your hair. Intensify a henna treatment by adding a still warm herbal rinse to the henna before applying.

To Spray or Not To Spray

If you find that your finished style requires a bit of extra holding power, use a little spray. Spritz sparingly, though. Organically beautiful hair does not equal helmet head. Also, look for pump sprays and stay away from aerosols. Aerosols introduce fine particles into your lungs and irritate them. You want hair sprays that have natural resinous ingredients like gum arabic, gum tragancanth, kava kava, nettles, potato starch, and turmeric. And look for products that contain panthenol, vitamins A and E, and wheat germ.

There are plenty of herbs to use in a color rinse. Try them to achieve some of these effects.

● A rinse of chamomile or calendula adds golden honey tones to blonde or light brown hair. Intensify the lightening action by adding lemon juice to the rinse and then drying your hair naturally in the sun. Rhubarb also imparts lovely golden yellow tones.

● Hibiscus accentuates red highlights in blonde, brown, or red hair.

● Sandalwood emphasizes reddish brown tones.

● Rosemary, sage, and strongly brewed tea or coffee all bring out deep brown tones.

● Indigo or elderberry intensify bluish black tones in brown or black hair.

if you do color...

Remember this advice for keeping colored hair as healthy as possible:

☐ Protect and condition your hair and scalp regularly.
☐ Don't stray far from your natural level and tone. Dramatic color changes require more upkeep, since outgrowth becomes very obvious very soon. (This reasoning also applies to texture services.)
☐ Follow your stylist's recommendations for a home-care regimen.
☐ Color-enhancing shampoos do work, helping you hold on to your desired color between salon or at-home color treatments, so do try them out.
☐ Be especially vigilant about protecting chemically treated and naturally colored hair from the sun.
☐ The less you chemically process your hair, the more healthy it remains.

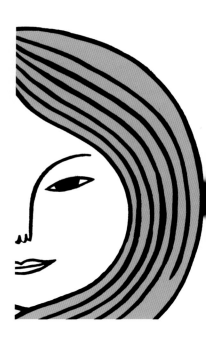

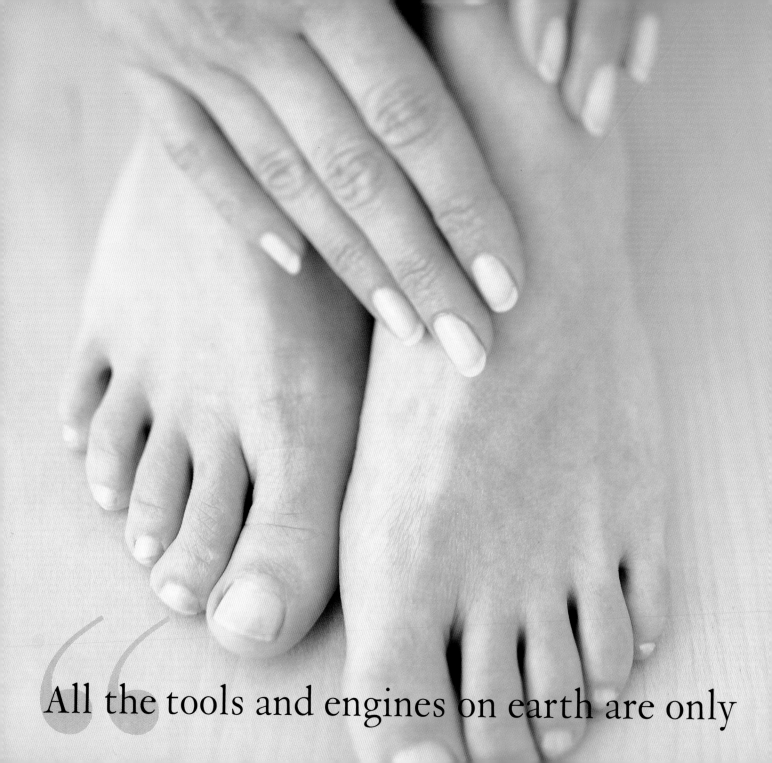

"All the tools and engines on earth are only

beautiful

feet, hands, and nails

extensions of [the body's] limbs and senses.

Ralph Waldo Emerson

Our hands and feet put us in **physical** touch with the world. Give your hands and feet proper love and attention, and you'll make your whole body feel good. Reflexology and accupressure give us an intimate understanding of this connection. We can affect **vitality** within every organ and gland, and the energy of our bodies, when we know how and where to touch specific areas on the palms of the hands and the soles of the feet. In fact, **massage** therapy for these wonderful and loyal body parts is so important that we will review specific applications for each. ● Two additional areas that universally affect your hands and feet include nutrition and **moisturizing**. I'll also cover the importance of a nutritionally balanced diet to protect the skin, which of course covers your hands and feet and ultimately promotes healthy cellular turnover, as well as **regeneration**. And on the subject of moisturizing hands and feet, I say, let yourself become addicted. Your hands, feet, and nails will look better, and it also just plain feels great. ● This chapter offers the essence of what it takes to maintain **beautiful** extremities. Give your hands, feet, and nails everything they require, so they can continue providing you with devoted service throughout a lifetime of organic experiences!

Organic Foot Care

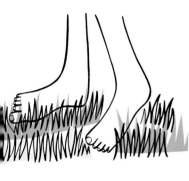

Leonardo da Vinci described feet as a masterpiece of engineering and a work of art. Organically speaking, our feet keep us grounded to the Earth's energies while also taking us where we want to go. Ah, what faithful servants our feet are! It's only fitting that we treat them with the care and attention they so richly deserve.

To understand what your feet need, it's probably best to first understand what makes a foot function. The human foot contains 26 bones, 33 joints, 19 muscles, and 107 ligaments. Virtually supporting the entire body, feet tend to hold or reflect the state of your mind and heart. If you don't believe me, consider the seemingly endless foot metaphors we use to describe our moods and inclinations. When we're decisive, self-confident, flexible, and on the move, we're fleet of foot or quick on our feet. When immobilized, weak, or wishy-washy, we have feet of clay or we're dragging our feet. We get a foot up on our business competitors, and our dogs howl after a long day of rushing around. So to put your best foot forward, start taking care of those feet today.

Keep the Blood Flowing

It's a long way from your heart to the tips of your toes, but for healthy, comfortable feet, it's important to encourage blood circulation to this area. Exercise and massage both play a role. In addition, you always want to choose well-fitting shoes. Forfeiting comfort for style might look great but the repercussions will have you walking down a painful path, possibly filled with bunions, calluses, or deformed toes.

Foot Exercises

Exercise is essential for maintaining the mobility and flexibility of your feet. Foot exercises may also relieve soreness, particularly if your problem is flat feet. Here are a few exercises that can be done anywhere, any time.

"But is it not sweet, with nimble feet, to

- Rock back and forth from your heels to your toes for several minutes.

- Try picking up marbles with your toes.

- Lay a towel flat on the floor, then scrunch your toes up on the towel and draw the fabric toward you.

- Roll your arches over a tennis ball, golf ball, or rolling pin.

Foot Massage

Massage, another treat for your feet, encourages better blood flow to this vital area and just plain feels good. As I described in "The Nature of Skin" on page 31, massaging your feet every night before bed induces profound relaxation. When you release tension in your feet, your mind-body physiology is certain to follow. Use a small amount of certified organic plant oil with 2 or 3 drops of geranium, lavender, patchouli, or tea tree essential oil, all of which possess potent antibacterial effects. You can find these ingredients in many store-bought preparations. If you prefer, make your own foot massage treatment by mixing 40 drops of any of these essential oils, alone or in combination, with 4 ounces of organic witch hazel. You can also add these aromatic essential oils to unscented lotion, introducing an element of aromatherapy to your foot massage.

Begin your massage by distributing your chosen massage oil or lotion over the palms of your hands. Briskly stroke the soles of the feet, then go on to massage the rest of the foot with a combination of small circular motions. Use longer strokes between the bones along the top of the foot, working toward the heel, and thus toward your heart. This is important for directing blood flow. Gently pull each toe outward from the base to the tip. Put on organic-cotton socks, and it's time for bed! You can do this every night for the rest of your life. It's a healthful part of your daily routine, and your feet will be absolutely beautiful to behold.

dance upon the air.
Oscar Wilde

How beautiful are the feet of them that…

Serve Your Feet Some Sole Food

A wide variety of feet treats will help soften rough and dry skin and invigorate or soothe your feet. A good old pumice stone is great on callused or rough skin. Use one in the shower after moistening your skin. Put a small amount of organic body wash on the stone and gently rub the callused area. Make sure you slather on a moisturizer afterward.

Another remedy for rough, callused foot skin is adding about 1 to 2 cups—the more the better—of pineapple juice to a footbath. An enzyme (called bromelain) in the juice naturally sloughs off dry skin. Or, you can try mixing 1 tablespoon of sea salt with 1 tablespoon of sweet almond oil. Soak, then scrub callused areas for a few minutes after your shower. Rinse, towel off, moisturize, and then don fluffy organic-cotton socks.

Warm Water Soak

Anytime your feet need a little TLC, give them a warm water soak. You may also add Epsom or sea salts, which help soften the rough, dry patches of your skin. A soak can mobilize the elimination of any buildup of toxins in the delicate joints, reduce buildup of dead cellular tissue, and control bacteria. This all serves to soothe, smooth, protect, and stabilize your feet. In addition, it's a great preparatory step before massaging your feet. Rinse your feet before massaging with a nourishing foot cream or oil.

Exfoliating products specific for the feet are also good choices. Some of these even have ground pumice in them. Seek out organic products with botanicals and plant and essential oils. Look for these healing foot-care herbs: peppermint to cool off and revive stressed or hot feet; lavender for its wonderful soothing quality, as well as its antiseptic power; sage for its tremendous anti-inflammatory, antiseptic, and antibacterial benefits; and tea tree oil for its healing, antibacterial, and antiviral qualities.

Let Your Feet Breathe

Your feet have about 250,000 sweat glands, producing as much as 8 ounces of sweat a day. This is why it's so important to wear sensible shoes that let your feet breathe. You'll also want to avoid

bring glad tidings of good things!

Romans 10:15

harsh cleansers or sprays that attempt to block or stop foot perspiration. This perspiration is your body's healthy, natural way of eliminating toxins.

If excessive perspiration is a problem, there are organic ways to balance the situation without hampering your body's ability to purge toxins.

- Make yourself a footbath by adding 2 to 6 drops of essential oil to a container filled with warm water. A few essential oils to try include eucalyptus, juniper, lavender, rosemary, and tea tree. These oils offer a combination of soothing or stimulating effects (see "Choosing Essential Oils" on page 103), as well as antiseptic and toning astringency qualities. Toning astringency acts to somewhat firm foot skin tissue and thus slightly reduce the amount of oil and perspiration excreted from the skin. The end results will be to balance the amount of foot perspiration expelled, wash sweat away, and refresh your feet. Of course, a footbath also leaves your feet smelling nice!

- Change your stockings or socks frequently.

- Drink at least 64 ounces of purified water each day, and even more if you are physically active, live in a particularly warm environment, or perspire a lot.

- Soak your feet in a bath that's been infused with black tea. Brew 2 tea bags in 2 pints of water, then add 2 quarts of cool water. The tannic acid acts as a drying agent and helps prevent odor.

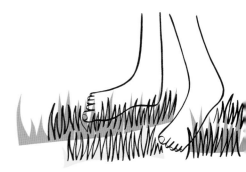

Organic Hand Care

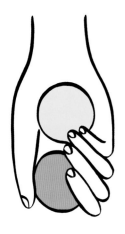

Your sense of touch is largely experienced through your hands—while giving yourself or your loved one a massage, running your hands through your loved one's hair, hugging someone dear, petting the glossy fur of a dog, feeling the silky touch of your bathrobe. I could think of enough examples to fill a page.

Life flows from our hands into action, as extensions of our heart center, and they carry out all of our heartfelt desires. As messengers of our emotions, they help us express our love. As extensions of our work, they perform a staggering amount of functional duties. Our hands are incredibly sensitive and distinctive. Your fingerprint belongs to you and you alone. Your palm displays your heart, head, and life lines, and hence your destiny. The hand, in a sense, has become symbolic of the whole body. Going a step further, spiritualists see the hand as a direct energetic connection to your soul and psyche.

Hand Yoga

Our hands work very hard for us, and after a long day on the job, they can become quite achy. It's as if each of the hand's 27 small bones, 30 joints, and 37 muscles are all crying for help. If we don't address these little pains, we could be looking at bigger problems later on, such as arthritis, tendonitis, carpal tunnel syndrome, and a variety of other repetitive stress injuries. If any part of your body deserves the white-glove treatment, it's your hands.

Just as we warm up our muscles before launching into full-body exercise, think about warming up and stretching your hands before beginning your day. Try to stretch your hands throughout the day, and stay mindful of how you sit and stand. Hand discomfort may sometimes be the result of poor posture, putting a strain on our back, neck, and shoulders, and finally our arms, hands, and fingers. Carpal tunnel syndrome, for example, is a swelling of the tunnel just below the wrist, and this swelling pinches the median nerve as it passes through the wrist. Often this is caused by repetitive movement and unnatural or awkward posturing. or when vertebrae in the neck become misaligned.

"The bird of paradise alights only upon the hand

The best way to prevent carpal tunnel syndrome is to be vigilant about changing the position of your body and hands when doing repetitive tasks. You also want to take stretch breaks every 10 to 15 minutes. Doing a few healthy hand stretches throughout the day is a good idea as well. Here are several exercises to get you moving.

- Interlock your fingers, palms facing away from you, and stretch your arms as far out as they will go. Feel the lovely stretch throughout your hands and arms. Stretch your wrists and arms.

- Chinese Harmony Balls—also called health spheres—help reduce stress and also stimulate your hand's acupressure points, muscles, and nerves. They also help improve blood circulation and energy flow, which in turn build strength and flexibility. Place these two balls in your hand and revolve them as long and as fast as you want. Focus your mind on the wonderfully melodic sound they make.

- Grip-strengthener balls provide many of the same benefits that Chinese Harmony Balls do. Keep them in your desk drawer, next to your bed or television, and in your car. They are great for stress relief and for developing hand and forearm strength. This is something simple that really works, but you do need to make a small commitment, taking a minute here and there throughout the day.

You can also try the following hand yoga sequence for maintaining a full range of motion.

1. _Place your right elbow on a flat surface_, with your right palm facing you.
2. _Place the left wrist in the right palm._ Let gravity take over as your left arm hangs there.
3. _Breathe deeply several times_, then gently arch your right wrist up, in the opposite direction it was hanging. This counterposes the first powerful stretch.

that does not grasp.
John Berry

My Carpal Tunnel Remedy

When I first began suffering from carpal tunnel syndrome, I found that the most effective treatment included a combination of chiropractic adjustments; vitamin B$_6$ therapy; and aromatherapy massages of the arm, wrist, and hand. The massage oil I selected was a mix of eucalyptus, lavender, and marjoram—10 drops of each—and 1 ounce of sweet almond oil. I massaged this into my hands and arms twice a day. Years later, none of the discomfort has returned. Of course, I still maintain the massages, and I always make sure to get the recommended daily allowance of vitamin B$_6$.

If you're presently dealing with any debilitating hand or wrist conditions, talk to your doctor before performing specific exercises.

4. *Repeat this sequence on the other side*, with your left hand supporting your right wrist.

5. *Next, again place your right elbow* on a flat surface with your palm facing toward you.

6. *Using your index and middle fingers* on your left hand, hang onto the thumb of your right hand.

7. *Take several deep breaths.* Bend your right fingers inward to counterstretch.

8. *Repeat this sequence* on the other side to stretch your left wrist.

These two stretches, performed together at intervals throughout the day, benefit strained tendons and muscles through the wrist.

Be Gentle to Your Hands

We all want silky, youthful hands, and you can have them if you'll simply give your hands a little of your time. Naturally, getting the dietary nutrients that encourage overall healthy skin and cellular turnover is the important first step. The next step is to make sure you get enough exercise, so that the nutrients you consume are properly delivered to the skin. These are both internal steps to protect your hands. Externally, there are things you can do as well. For one, you want to protect your hands—both the skin and nails—from dehydrating and potentially discoloring elements. Keep natural handwashing liquid and nourishing moisturizer at every sink in the house. Carry a small container of moisturizer with you. While you're working the moisturizer in, give yourself a mini hand massage. Stroke, gently roll, and milk the fingers from base to fingertip. This eases the joints. Massage with small circular strokes through the palm area. Rub the thumb, apply pressure to the web between each finger, then move on to the soft tissue between the tendons and bones on the back of your hand, moving toward your wrist. This is all about increasing blood and energy flow.

Make it a habit to moisturize your hands often during the day and especially before bed! This is the most effective way to preserve and shield your hands from environmental stressors.

Here are a few more strategies to keep your hands happy and healthy:

● Have a professional hand treatment in tandem with a manicure. Professional manicurists or massage therapists often offer arm- and hand-massage treatments that are relaxing as well as beautifying.

● A soak in sea salt can be quite helpful if your hands are swollen or sore. For a sea salt soak, see "Natural Masks and Exfoliants" on page 52.

● For hands as smooth as silk, soak them in warm milk for 5 to 10 minutes. You can do this once a week if desired. You can also use calendula and chamomile essential oils to nourish and moisturize the skin of your hands—by adding 2 or 3 drops to either a warm water hand soak or to the hand lotion or plant oil you use to moisturize and massage your hands.

● Smear organic honey, one of nature's best moisturizers, over your hands and relax for 10 to 15 minutes. When you're through relaxing, wash your hands with a gentle soap and warm water.

● Be sure to use your body exfoliating product on your hands, as well. You want to encourage the sloughing off of dead skin cells and cellular turnover here, too.

In general, many of the skin treatments that I described in "The Nature of Skin" (see page 31) will be very beneficial for the skin of your hands.

Remember Those Gloves

When heading outdoors, don't forget to protect your hands from the elements. Be sure to apply a hand lotion and overall body sunscreen of at least SPF 15, and if you're headed out to the garden or out and about on a cold day, be sure to wear gloves. And don't forget the gloves when washing dishes. In addition to protection, gloves can also serve to increase your hand moisturizer's effect. Before bed, try this trick: Moisturize your hands and then slip into soft, comfy, lightweight, organic cotton gloves. When you awake in the morning, your hands will be softer than ever imagined.

Organic Nail Care

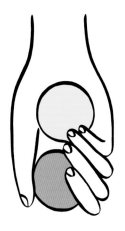

Defining your fingers and toes are your nails. There's no denying the beauty of healthy nails, but they also serve a wonderful purpose, providing 20 tough and protective protein plates that guard our fingertips. Our nails are made from the same keratin protein as our hair.

Like your skin and hair, your nails will richly benefit from a whole foods organic diet. Get plenty of fruits and vegetables, complex carbohydrates, and protein. Make sure you take in the recommended daily requirements of the essential nail vitamins and minerals, including vitamin A or the vegetable precursor beta carotene, all the vitamin Bs, vitamin C, calcium, magnesium, zinc, and silica. Get essential fatty acids from your diet or through supplements. And for goodness' sake, wean yourself off of junk food, sweets, and sodas. Remember what Hippocrates said: "Let food be your medicine, and medicine be your food." Our body is a direct reflection of the food we eat. You will be amazed at the difference in your nails, skin, and hair—not to mention your overall sense of well-being—once you eliminate foods that don't contribute to your overall health.

It is interesting to note that in many traditional health approaches, one's nails are said to indicate a variety of health conditions. For example, red, blue, yellow, or any other strange discoloration of your nails can be a sign of disease or other medical problem.

If you're concerned about any unusual condition of your nails, don't try to self-diagnose: See your doctor.

Beauty Nailed Down

For lovely nails, you want to begin as you do with the hands—moisturize! With moisture, your nails and surrounding skin will maintain a more lustrous, soft, and resilient look. Any moisturizer or plant oil worked into your hands can be used to massage your nails, as well. Alternate with treatments that contain AHAs to optimize the sloughing off of dead cellular tissue and retention of moisture in your nail bed and cuticle area.

Here's a hand, nail, and cuticle oil mixture that I find very nutritive and moisturizing. Add a few drops of carrot seed oil, rose, or rosewood essential oil to ½ ounce of sesame oil and ½ ounce of grapeseed oil. The carrot seed oil smells yummy and helps strengthen the nails. The rose and rosewood oils are both moisturizing and have a wonderful, exotic aroma!

Another mixture begins by combining sea salt with pulverized (use your blender or coffee grinder) dried lavender, or rosebuds, or both, plus a mixture of citrus peels—orange, grapefruit, and tangerine. All these ingredients should be in equal parts, and quantities should be determined by the finished amount you feel you need. Add to enough purified water to create an organic herbal sea-salt scrub for the hands that is nutritive, moisturizing, and very efficient for sloughing off dead cellular tissue. You can also float these ingredients in a hand- or footbath to soothe, relax, and moisturize your skin, nails, and cuticles.

Manicures and Pedicures

A gentle manicure or pedicure can be quite soothing, whether it's done by yourself in the comfort of your own home or by a trained specialist in a spa environment. When you add a relaxing hand-and-arm or foot-and-leg massage, the benefits are especially wonderful. When indulging in such luxury, strive for an organic approach to beautiful nails. Many typical products used on fingernails and toenails contain harmful chemicals (some of which

Don't Get Hung Up on Hangnails

Hangnails are a nuisance. These rough slivers of detached skin snag on everything, from clothing to pantyhose, and can become downright painful. To avoid hangnails, wear gloves whenever washing dishes or doing housecleaning. Regular moisturizing goes a long way toward alleviating hangnails, too. Lotions with aloe, calendula, and comfrey are particularly healing. You can also soak your fingertips in lukewarm comfrey tea. The comfrey contains allantoin, a constituent with cellular regenerative properties.

To mix your own nail and cuticle oil, combine ½ ounce of organic plant oil, ¼ teaspoon of vitamin E oil, and 1 or 2 drops each of lavender and frankincense essential oils. Work this into your nails and cuticles every morning and night until the hangnails subside. Not only is this antiseptic, but it smells heavenly, too!

are possible carcinogens) or ingredients that just smell downright offensive. By seeking treatments that bow to the calming properties of aromatherapy and by selecting toxin-free products that naturally enrich the nails, you won't undo all the delightful benefits of a manicure and pedicure.

Growing Pains

There's nothing more painful than an infected ingrown toenail. Okay, maybe there are more painful conditions, but when suffering from this ailment, it's hard to imagine anything worse. To prevent ingrown toenails, wear shoes that fit well, especially if your nails tend to grow in a downward curve along the outer edges. Make sure you trim your toenails straight across.

Soaking your feet can soothe an ingrown nail and help ward off infection. Tea tree oil and grapefruit seed extract are both quite effective. You can use anywhere from 10 to 15 drops of tea tree oil in your footbath. Some experts also recommend taking the homeopathic remedy Silicea 6X orally 3 times a day until the ingrown nail improves. This treatment is derived from silica (crystalline in nature and a good conductor of the life force energy), an element found abundantly in nature. It is excellent for supporting the skin's connective tissue and the growth of hair and nails, especially given their crystalline properties. Silicea tends to strengthen the nail and encourage it to grow straight.

While manicures and pedicures are wonderfully relaxing and make our hands and feet look and feel great, they can lead to fungal and bacterial infections if certain precautions are not taken. If you give yourself manicures and pedicures or visit a local spa to have these services done, make sure proper hygiene rules are followed, that all instruments are properly sterilized, and that all equipment and solutions are of the highest quality. Make sure tools and solutions are either fresh or properly cleaned before touching you. Antiseptic solutions and micro-wave sterilizers are believed to adequately kill germs, but some women go a step further and bring their own equipment to the salon or spa.

If you're susceptible to dry, brittle, flaking nails, try taking a break from nail polish, since conventional nail polishes tend to aggravate these conditions. When you remove polish, always use a nonacetone nail polish remover. It's also wise to use polishes that are formaldehyde and toluene free—toluene is found in adhesives, and recent tests suggest that this chemical may be carcinogenic. You might also consider some of the wonderful organic strengthening polishes and nail treatments available today.

If your nails are healthy but look bad due to temporary staining from nail polishes, try soaking them for 10 minutes in a mixture of equal parts hydrogen peroxide and warm water. Then gently brush each nail with a nail brush, using a paste of baking soda and water. It works like a charm!

Cuticle Care

As for your cuticles, remember that they protect the nail matrix from dirt and bacteria. (The nail matrix describes the active tissue that generates cells, which harden as they move outward from the root to the nail.) Since the matrix involves live tissue and cells, it is vital that you treat this area kindly! Gently tend to the nail matrix and keep it moisturized and healthy. Don't cut your cuticles or aggressively push them back. (This goes for hands as well as feet.) Instead, gently push them back with a moist towel. A cotton swab also works well. I like to gently push my cuticles back with my thumbnail as I shower. Apply a penetrating oil to your cuticles after coming out of the shower. Avocado, canola, grapeseed, jojoba, and sesame oil are good choices, since these plant oils have deeper absorption capabilities because of the size of their molecules. Skip this step, or at least rinse completely afterward, if you plan to apply polish. And never use a pointy tool to clean under your nails. This can cause infection or even cut your nail. Instead, use a soft nail brush to gently clean under your nails—another great step to do in the shower.

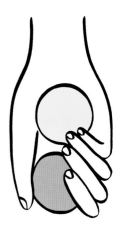

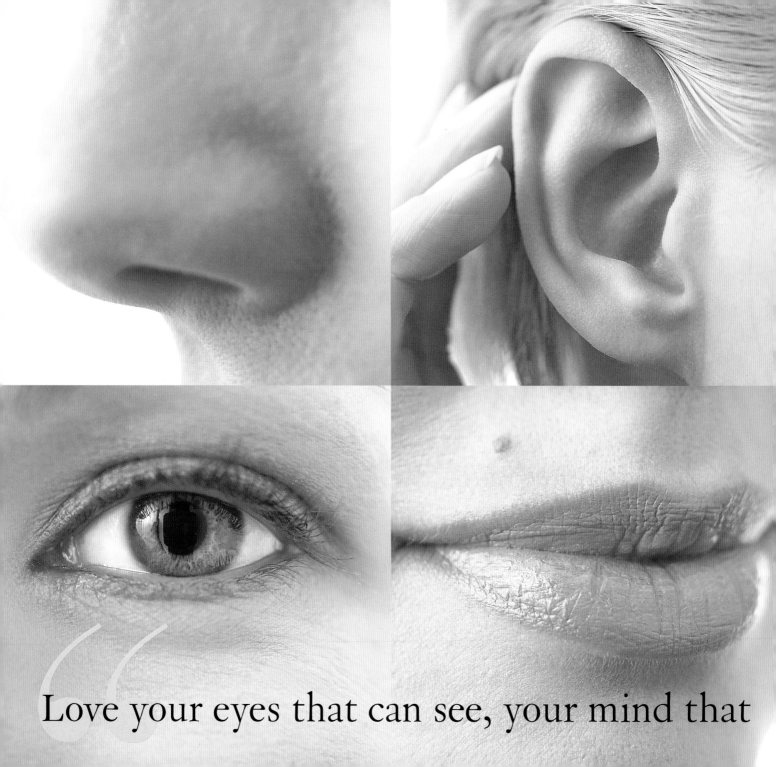

Love your eyes that can see, your mind that

organic beauty
for the senses

can hear the music, the thunder of wings.
(John) Robinson Jeffers

Your **senses** are the gateway to your consciousness. Your outer environment melds with your inner environment to profoundly affect your mind-body physiology. If you are feeling discomfort, uneasiness, or imbalance of any kind, you can use your five senses to create great healing and **pacifying** influences for your nervous system, as well as the energy field that surrounds you. Your five senses will serve you just as remarkably if you simply want to tap into the expansiveness of your mind, body, and **spirit**. Yet sometimes we forget how to do all these things. I suggest you take a moment and look within. ● Deep down inside, you know the difference between healthful and harmful as they pertain to your body. Tap into the nourishing wisdom that is inherent within you. You know what is best for you. Exercise. Nutrition. **Sleep**. Stress relief. They are integral to the optimum functioning of your faculties. These practices keep your immune system humming along in top form and keep you **sensually** tuned in. It is so easy today to disregard and neglect your five senses through cumulative and mindless actions. I urge you to witness what you do and surround yourself with a world that is touching, easy on the eye, tasty, music to the ears, and heavenly **fragrant**. You're nurturing the life force—this is organic beauty at its best!

"Beholding beauty with the eye of the mind…

Eye Candy

As Dante said, "Thence we came forth to see the stars." Our eyes allow us to feast on the beauty of colors, textures, and patterns surrounding us, which in turn helps to create a better balance in our mind-body physiology. For people with normal vision, the majority of the sensory information the brain receives registers through the eyes.

To heighten the mind-body balance, I try to minimize exposure to graphic violence, whether in the newspaper or on television. Seeing and hearing about murder and mayhem can have detrimental effects on your health, creating depression and raising stress levels. Instead of viewing media-sponsored violence, I prefer to walk in nature and watch the miracle of life unfolding. To mingle and dance with the rhythms of nature on a regular basis is good for the heart and soul. If you don't have the opportunity to literally join nature, try visualizing a wonderful place in your mind. It's all eye candy—a sweet treat for the mind, body, and soul.

Take It Easy on Your Eyes

While visualized nature walks may be perfectly focused, our literal eyesight can sometimes make real strolls through life appear somewhat fuzzy. So how can you keep your eyes from becoming tired or strained and thus hold on to better vision? Don't work at computers, don't read books, don't watch television, and don't sit in classrooms. Do spend lots of time in nature, gazing into the distance. Okay—I know these suggestions are not the most realistic. Instead I urge everyone to begin protecting their eyesight with regular eye exams, minimal exposure to environmental allergens and toxins, lots of exercise, plenty of rest, and maximum attention to proper nutrition. Did you know that more than 25 percent of the nutrients

bring[s] forth, not images of beauty, but realities.

Plato

we absorb from our food go to nourish our visual system? Alone or in combination, these steps help stave off wrinkled skin, puffiness, and dark circles around the eyes. They also strengthen the body's ability to naturally thwart eyestrain and eyesight deficiencies.

To counter eyestrain, do the following:

● Practice stress reduction, meditation, and viewing beautiful visual treats. All of these are of paramount importance when resting your mind and in turn, your eyes. Here are some ways to relax your optic nerve, enhance blood circulation, and relieve muscular tension in and around your eyes: Tighten your eye muscles by squeezing your eyes tightly shut, then gently open your eyes, letting tension dissolve away. Blink several times as you turn your head from side to side. Remember to breathe deeply though each phase of this exercise. Focus on objects at varying distances at regular intervals throughout the day to give your eyes a break. "Palm" your eyes—briskly rub your palms together and then place them over your closed eyes. Relax as you pay attention to your breathing for a few moments. Do any and all of these several times a day.

● Treat yourself to daily serenity checks, where you soften and relax your facial features. To do this, gently close your eyes and consciously let your muscles relax. Make sure there's no furrowed brow, no frowning or even smiling, no scrunched-tight eyes. Just let the muscles hang. This is a very conscious part of witnessing tension that is held in certain parts of the face and body and in

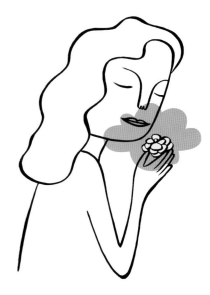

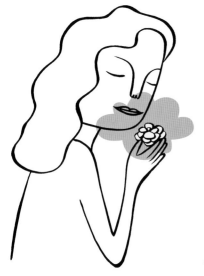

turn telling yourself to release these held tensions. It's not an exercise as much as it's a serenity check-in.

● Keep the lachrymal glands, or tear ducts, in optimal working condition. This is vital for washing away debris or bacteria that touches your eyeball. If you are experiencing severe or persistent dry eyes, see your doctor. You may need artificial tears, either by prescription or over the counter. Either way, you should use a preservative-free treatment. Temporary problems may be remedied with the organic eyewash treatment on page 98.

To help protect your eyesight in general, try these activities.

● Ingest burdock, dandelion, and milk thistle cleansers in herbal form; they're all wonderful detoxifiers for the liver and blood.

● Eliminate or cut down on fatty foods, simple refined sugars, salt, coffee, alcohol, and carbonated beverages.

Eye Yoga

Regular eye-area massages and a few simple eye exercises performed throughout the day can help relax, cleanse, and strengthen your eyes. To massage the eye area, use an organic oil, such as sweet almond oil, and with your ring fingers, gently press around your eye socket from the outer corner, along the bottom edge, and then along the top of your eyelid, just below the brow bone. Repeat this several times, preferably right before bed.

Try this simple exercise to strengthen the muscles used to focus your eyes: Hold a finger about 1 foot away from your face, at nose level, and focus on it for 10 seconds.

Now shift your focus to an object about 10 feet away, again focusing for 10 seconds. This is one round. Do 10 rounds of this exercise, then relax. You can do this several times throughout the day.

Eye Nourishment

Your eyes depend on the vitamins, minerals, and protein that you get from eating a variety of foods. Eat plenty of fruits and vegetables, particularly the yellow- and orange-color varieties, such as sweet potatoes and winter squash. You also want to eat plenty of poultry, fish, nuts, seeds, and whole grains. Keep your intake of saturated animal fats and salt to a minimum. Get enough of the antioxidants vitamin C and vitamin E. Vitamin D, iron, copper, zinc, calcium, and protein all play significant roles in the health of your eyes, as well. Herbs for eyes include eyebright and bilberry. Both herb supplements are easily found in whole foods or herb stores.

Eye Cleansing

I don't recommend commercial eyedrops, but suggest one of the following eye treatments instead. When applied over closed eyes for 15 to 20 minutes, each serves a delicious and soothing purpose.

- Cotton pads doused with ice cold organic milk and placed over the eyes in the morning help reduce puffiness.

- Cotton pads damp with rosewater help soothe bloodshot eyes.

- Cucumber, apple, or potato slices soothe and reduce puffiness.

- Cooled black tea bags provide a strong astringent that shrinks swollen tissues and thus reduces puffiness.

Computer Vision Syndrome

People working at computers blink much less than they do when at rest. You normally blink up to 22 times each minute, but in front of a computer, that number drops to just 7 times each minute. This can result in eye fatigue and irritation, blurred or double vision, as well as headaches. To combat these consequences, blink regularly when you're doing computer work. Every 20 to 30 minutes, redirect your focus to objects at different distances. Make sure the top of your computer screen is at eye level and a full arm's distance away. Also, make sure you have proper lighting. Finally, consider purchasing a computer screen filter, which may help protect your eyes from glare.

● Chilled chamomile tea bags or compresses soothe and reduce swelling. To make a compress, put 2 tablespoons of the herb into 1 cup of water; boil, cool, and strain. Dip cotton pads or a washcloth (chamomile will stain) into the tea, and place over your eyes.

● A warm calendula tea compress soothes eye irritation. You make a compress by dipping a washcloth or small cotton pads in brewed and cooled calendula tea, then placing the washcloth or cotton pads against your eyes. Calendula tea bags—steeped and then cooled— may also be used instead of a compress.

● A cold water compress helps relieve itchy eyes.

Using an Eyewash

To wash your eyes, you may purchase a prepared organic eyewash or make your own by boiling 2 tablespoons of dried organic eyebright in 16 ounces of purified water. Cool, then strain. Fill an eyecup, then apply it over your eye and blink for up to 30 seconds. If you don't have an eyecup, you may also put a cotton pad, saturated with the eyewash, over your eyes and lie down for 15 to 20 minutes. Dried eyebright is available at most health food stores.

When allergies create watery, itchy, irritated eyes, consider quercetin, a bioflavonoid that blocks the flood of histamines, substances that the body releases when exposed to allergy triggers. Again, you can generally find quercetin in health food stores.

You Look Marvelous

When it comes to what you put in and around your eyes—such as makeup or contact lenses—you want to be particularly careful. Your eyes are extremely sensitive, and a little care up front can prevent all sorts of possible problems later—from nasty bacterial infections to temporary allergic reactions.

● If you wear contacts, consider using a natural, preservative-free contact lens solution. You can readily find this type of product at most stores that carry organic product lines.

● Be careful with eye makeup. Throw out any makeup that is 6 months old—discarding it after 3 months is even better. Look for hypoallergenic eye makeup formulas. There are organic eye makeup product lines, but you will probably have better luck finding products containing mostly natural ingredients and at least some organic ingredients.

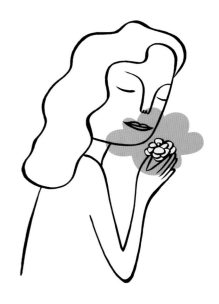

● Use organic almond, olive, or jojoba oils to gently massage the eye area, or use these oils on a dampened cotton pad to gently remove eye makeup.

● Each night, use a cotton swab to brush a light application of olive or castor oil along your brows and lashes. Over time this creates thicker, more lustrous lashes and brows.

● Always wear sunglasses with ultraviolet protection when you're in bright sunlight.

● Stop smoking! Smoking creates wrinkles around your eyes.

The Nose Knows

Your nose, situated smack in the middle of your face, is yet another miracle of creation. Your sense of smell has the ability to bring back pleasurable memories, calm emotions, and wipe away stress. Your nose really does know!

In addition to its emotional powers, your nose also possesses great physical powers. As you breathe in and out through your nose, mucous membranes block bacteria and dust particles from entering the body. Nose hairs warm the air entering your lungs and prevent a perpetual runny nose by keeping mucous secretions toward the back of your throat. To keep these natural processes happening, it's important to maintain an immune system capable of staving off head colds or sinusitis. When the inevitable stuffy nose does come your way, a vaporizer or steam with eucalyptus, juniper, or tea tree

Soft is the music that would charm forever;

essential oils can help clear things up. However, if you're plagued by nasal polyps, a deviated septum, or any other malady that prevents you from breathing normally through your nose, seek proper medical attention.

Aromatherapy

Every time you experience an aroma, a river of emotions and memories is unleashed—feelings from desire to disgust—depending on your brain's response to that one smell. Tapping into this enormous power is the science of aromatherapy, where scents—often beginning with but not restricted to essential oils—are used to treat the mind-body physiology. These essential oils are the subtle, aromatic, and volatile life force energy extracted from different tree and bush flowers, seeds, leaves, stems, bark, roots, fruits, and herbs. Whether you enjoy a particular oil by inhaling its airborne scent or by applying the oil directly onto your skin, molecules from this essential oil enter into your bloodstream and offer the body hundreds of powerful natural chemical constituents that nurture your physical, mental, emotional, and spiritual balance. You may think that positively impacting your physical and emotional well-being just by sniffing some oil sounds too good to be true, but there are many studies out right now that confirm the mood-enhancing and therapeutic qualities of essential oils.

Inhaling the scent of an essential oil affects your mind, mood, and emotions. This process also releases hormones to your organs and body cells. Reactions can be calming, cooling, invigorating, or stimulating. When applied externally, the essential oil molecules affect the body—skin, muscles, joints, and organs—by penetrating the skin, entering the dermal layer, and interacting with blood and lymph vessels, connective tissue, sebaceous and sweat glands, sensory nerves, and hair follicles. The positive effects run the gamut, including moisturizing the skin, balancing the mind-body

The flower of sweetest smell is shy and lowly.

William Wordsworth

physiology, calming the emotions, and acting as an anti-inflammatory for body tissues. Essential oils can also promote elimination of waste matter and regeneration of new cells.

Essential oils can vary tremendously in their quality and cost, but this is an area where you don't want to compromise. Make sure your essential oils are from a reputable company, are certified organic, and are from 100 percent pure essential oils—with no suspenders, synthetic dilutants, or mineral oil. Marketers have jumped on the aromatherapy bandwagon, and you'll see lots of wanna-bes out there. These fake products often contain artificial fragrances and artificial colors that can potentially cause allergic reactions.

Essential Aromatherapy Instructions

While aromatherapy involves any scent that triggers welcome emotions, the science most often begins by selecting an essential oil that encourages a specific positive response. To best understand and use essential oils, visit your local health food store or whole foods market. Go through the samplers to discover how the different essential oils resonate with you. You'll instinctively be drawn to your favorites. To begin, choose one that is calming, such as lavender, chamomile, melissa, or patchouli, and one that is stimulating, such as peppermint or grapefruit. You may use these in a variety of ways:

- Mix several drops into 1 ounce of organic plant oil and massage your feet, scalp, or any area that needs love and attention.

- Mist the air that surrounds you. You can do this by mixing a few drops of essential oil with purified water in an atomizer, or you can use a floral water. Usually sold in a spray bottle, floral water is the byproduct of the steamed distillation method that creates essential oils.

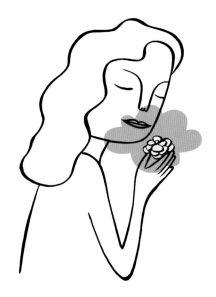

● At the start of the wash cycle, put a few drops of essential oil in the washing machine, along with your detergent. A few drops will not stain, and after the rinse cycle, just a faint hint of the wonderful aroma will remain.

● Use a vaporizer or diffuser to float oils into your environment. Try eucalyptus and juniper in the bedroom at night if you have a stuffy head, lavender in the evening to calm jittery nerves, or citrus oils in the morning to get going.

● Place a small clay diffuser with essential oils in your automobile. This can produce a profoundly positive and calming effect, especially when caught in traffic. For a list of the most calming essential oils, see "Choosing Essential Oils" on the opposite page.

● Place a drop of oil on a cool light bulb. After you turn the light on, the bulb heats the fragrance and disperses it throughout the room. You can also purchase a ceramic diffuser that fits over the bulb. I especially like to do this when staying in a hotel.

● Add essential oils to your skin- and hair-care products to enhance their benefits and features and strengthen them. Or purchase organic personal care items that already contain pure essential oils.

● Take a bath with essential oils. First, put a few drops of your desired essential oil into a carrier oil. This will dilute the essential oil and prevent it from getting into your eyes as you bathe (which can be damaging to the eyes). Next, fill the tub and add your prepared oil mix. Do not put the oils in as the tub fills since this may cause the oil molecules to dissipate too quickly.

● Make smelling salts by placing 1 tablespoon of rock salt and 10 drops of basil, peppermint, or rosemary essential oil (or a mix of these) in a small container with a tight-fitting lid. Uncap and inhale as desired, stimulating clear thought and providing an instant pick-me-up.

● Scented candles are wonderful for meditation, relaxation, and special occasions. Make sure the candle is made with pure essential oils, natural beeswax, and a natural, nonlead wick.

Choosing Essential Oils

These are some of my favorite essential oils. Try them out, and use the books in "Recommended Reading and Resources" (see page 134) to explore other possibilities. As you experiment, you'll come up with your own list of best scents!

Basil. Spicy, sweet, and refreshing. It stimulates clear thinking and provides an instant pick-me-up.

Chamomile. Sweet, herbaceous, and fruity. It calms the nerves and heals dry, sensitive, or inflamed skin.

Clary sage. This herb is wonderful for a woman's dream work (work the mind accomplishes while asleep and dreaming). It also supports the cells and hormones, stimulates the body's natural production of estrogen, and helps with headaches, coughs, and dry or mature skin.

Eucalyptus. A fresh, powerful scent that is antiseptic and used for respiratory congestion. It also alleviates sorrow and clears the mind.

Geranium. Sweet and rosy, with fruity and minty undertones. It helps balance women's moods and skin.

Grapefruit. Made from the fruit's rind, this oil relieves respiratory congestion and revitalizes the spirit. Orange oil accomplishes much the same results.

Lavender. Sweet, balsamic, and herbaceous. This oil produces a relaxing scent and has analgesic, antiseptic, and anti-inflammatory properties.

> # If music be the food of love, play on.
> *William Shakespeare*

Peppermint. Uplifting, cooling, and refreshing. It soothes the digestion process, helps purify and balance, and is excellent with inflammatory skin conditions.

Rose. Uplifting, it stirs the creative and romantic spirit, gently stimulates circulation, and is simply the best choice for skin care.

Rosemary. Invigorating, it improves circulation and soothes overworked muscles. It also helps focus the mind.

Sandalwood. Exotic, warm, seductive, and distinctive. It is excellent for moisturizing and regenerating the skin.

Ylang-ylang. Considered an aphrodisiac. Coupled with rosemary or lavender, it is excellent for sleep. It's also good for balancing and moisturizing the skin.

Sound Advice

Our ears have tiny hairs within the fluid-filled inner ear. These hairs move when sound vibrations hit them, triggering electrical impulses to the brain, where sound is interpreted. Through the ages, these interpretations have been credited with great healing powers. It appears that certain sounds create a resonance within our nervous system and bring a balance to our mind-body physiology. Sounds trigger a variety of physical changes, altering skin temperature, brain-wave patterns, and levels of stress hormones in the bloodstream.

Good Vibrations

Music can calm, soothe, or energize. It has also been shown to alleviate stress, insomnia, and depression and improve concentration and memory, boost immunity, and reduce pain. I like to call music that has a slow tempo and is filled with violins and flutes that soothe my soul my "going-to-heaven" music. At the other end of the spectrum, there is stimulating music, live with horns and percussion that seem to exhilarate the mind and body.

Easy listening, opera, jazz, rock and roll, Latin rhythms, techno ambient, and yes, even hip-hop—they all have a power to enhance and balance your vitality and energies. Regardless of what your mood and personal preferences are, you want to listen from a comfortable sitting position, eyes closed, and breathing in a smooth, deep pattern. Go into the music with your body, mind, and soul. Whether the music is sedating or stimulating, follow your instincts and become one with the music. It's a wonderful way to meditate, pray, or go into trance. If the mood feels right, dance till you sweat. This is one of the most universal forms of self-healing—physical activity coming together with music to energize and invigorate the body and soul.

Hear This!

To further enhance your hearing powers, listen to your body and take action. If you experience a ringing or itching in your ears, you may have an earwax buildup or blockage. Try one of the following therapies. As always, consult with your doctor about any persistent problems with your ears or your hearing.

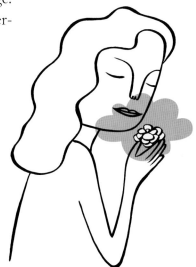

- Use an eyedropper to put a couple drops of hydrogen peroxide in each ear. Gently rinse your ear with a bulb ear syringe filled with warm water. Do this once a day for a couple of days.

- Lie on your side and place 10 warm drops of sesame oil in your ear canal. Pull your earlobe down to let the oil flow in. Rest in this position for 5 minutes. Then place a cotton ball in your ear, turn over, and repeat on the opposite side. Finish up by lying on your back for a few

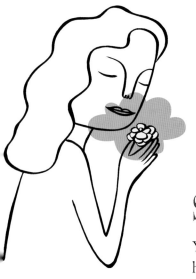

minutes. This treatment should be done in the early morning and no more than once a year. (Never put anything in your ear if you think your eardrum could have burst.)

● Reduce your intake of stimulants such as caffeine, tobacco, alcohol, aspirin, and tonic water—they're all thought to aggravate hearing problems.

Sink Your Teeth into This

Your mouth is the gateway to your entire body—everything that enters the mouth has the potential to help or harm. Your mouth—including your lips, teeth, gums, and tongue—is where the digestive process begins, and it is home to your sense of taste. There are 10,000 taste buds across the broad expanse of your tongue, and they distinguish sweet, sour, salty, pungent, bitter, and astringent flavors. Having a tongue allows you to talk to the world. Your lips are a provocative extension of the mucous membranes found inside the mouth. Your teeth express your happiness and pleasure when you flash your pearly whites. Your gums hold and support your teeth.

Lip Service

Highly sensitive, lips contain specialized sensors near the skin's surface that respond to the slightest stimulation. These sensors are found in but a few places on the body—on the lips and tongue, palms of the hands, soles of the feet, nipples, clitoris, and penis. Your lips do not have any melanin to protect them, unlike the rest of your body's skin, and they have no oil glands. These facts contribute to potential lip problems, such as burning, chapping, and dryness. So it's up to you to keep your lips as healthy as possible.

To protect your lips, you may want to try the following:

● Drink plenty of pure water to keep your lips moisturized from the inside out. Limit alcohol and caffeine, given their dehydrating qualities.

● Eat a balanced diet that provides the full spectrum of vitamins and minerals—particularly vitamin B and iron.

● Use organic lipsticks that get their pigment from natural sources such as iron oxides.

● Use a soft children's toothbrush to brush your lips. This removes dead skin and increases blood circulation to the area.

● Heal chapped lips with organic lip balms made from natural emollients like vegetable oils, natural waxes, or cocoa butter. In a pinch, use a dab of sweet almond or olive oil. When outdoors, make sure your lip balm has a sunscreen of at least SPF 15.

Don't Gum Up the Works

I've heard it said that the longer we keep our natural teeth, the longer our life span. Holding on to your original issue depends largely on the health of your gums. Genetics aside, problems with teeth and gums are generally rooted in oral hygiene. It really is important to brush, floss, and visit the dentist at least twice a year!

Brush, Brush, Brush

Always brush your teeth after eating. Use small circular motions, spending about 3 minutes on your full set of choppers. Dentists recommend soft, nylon bristles instead of

Have You Had Your Serving of Lipstick Today?

It is said that a woman can consume up to 4 pounds of lipstick in a lifetime. If you wear conventional lipsticks, there's a good chance you're ingesting potentially harmful ingredients. Because of this, many people consider lipstick to be one of the most toxic cosmetics available. There is the possibility of allergic reaction, as well as exposure to ingredients linked to certain cancers. These ingredients include Food, Drug, and Cosmetic (FD&C) and Drug and Cosmetic (D&C) dyes derived from coal tar, butylated hydroxyanisole (a preservative), and polyvinylpyrrolidone (a plastic resin). This complex issue involves ongoing governmental, scientific, and legal investigation. There remain enormous gray areas in what is acceptable and safe, probably exacerbated by the fact that the beauty industry is self-governing, and the FDA cosmetics office is truly dwarfed by the $36.4-plus billion cosmetics industry. So there are plenty of reasons to seek out natural and organic personal-care items.

Escape the Grind

Some people tend to grind their teeth when they're stressed. If you have this problem during stressful times, put your tongue either between your teeth or along the top of the mouth. This keeps your teeth apart, preventing you from grinding or tightening your jaw. Grinding your teeth during sleep can damage the jaw's musculoskeletal structure, as well as tooth enamel. Talk to your dentist about a tooth guard, or better yet, use stress-reduction techniques like meditation, yoga, and deep breathing.

natural bristles, which tend to be hard and injurious to the gums. Use natural herbal toothpastes, powders, and mouthwashes. Look for the following ingredients on product labels: bloodroot, echinacea, goldenseal, green tea, and myrrh.

You can make your own bacteria-fighting toothpaste and mouthwash by mixing a thick paste of baking soda and hydrogen peroxide. Add a drop of peppermint essential oil for taste. Follow with a rinse of 1 teaspoon of sea salt dissolved in 8 ounces of warm water. For a mouthwash, add a drop of peppermint essential oil to 1 ounce of water.

Also, use unwaxed floss for at least a minute or two every day. Look for natural flosses with cinnamon or tea tree oil, both good for their antibacterial properties.

Strawberries have a natural cleansing and bleaching effect, and they can provide a great alternative to brushing when you're camping. Crush a strawberry and gently massage the pulp over your teeth. Rinse afterward.

Saliva Is Important

A cleansing flow of saliva is important for good oral health, and a dry mouth promotes decay. If your saliva flow is negligible, if you're undergoing radiation treatments, or if you're using drugs that dry your mouth out, speak to your doctor. In addition to medicinal solutions, try sipping water throughout the day to keep yourself better hydrated.

Chewing gums made with parsley seed oil, sunflower oil, spearmint oil, or the natural sweetener xylitol can be beneficial in keeping a healthy saliva flow. Chewing these gums after every meal also helps flush away cavity-causing bacteria, sugars, and acids.

Nutrition Has Its Role

Of course, for healthy teeth, you don't want to eat tons of sugary foods that can lead to tooth decay. You do, however, want to eat a healthy, organic, unrefined diet including plenty of raw foods and roughage to help massage your gums. In addition, you want to get plenty of calcium and magnesium, either from your food or through supplements. Also make sure you're getting enough chromium, zinc, and selenium in your diet—all instrumental in keeping the natural cleansing fluids flowing to your teeth. Enhance your immune function with antioxidants—particularly vitamin C and CoQ_{10}.

Try a Massage for the Mouth

Massage can be as good for your mouth as it is for the rest of your body. Massage your gums every day. Place a small bit of olive or sesame oil on the pad of a finger and gently massage all gum surfaces. This is tremendous for stimulating healthy blood flow to the gums.

You can also activate blood and lymph circulation in your mouth and face muscles by exercising your face. Here are three good ways to do this.

- Twitch your noise back and forth.

- Puff your cheeks out and breathe deeply through your nose 10 times. Release and relax your cheeks.

- Stretch your mouth wide open, open your eyes all the way, and stick your tongue out as far as it will go. Release and relax.

For Better Breath

For fresh breath, try chewing on fennel seeds, parsley, or natural mints, or use a natural breath spray. Look for products containing cinnamon, echinacea, and peppermint to control bacteria while freshening the breath.

Scraping your tongue in the morning can also reduce bad breath and plaque because it eradicates bacteria buildup. Tongue scrapers are widely available these days. If you haven't tried one yet, pick one up at your local health food store.

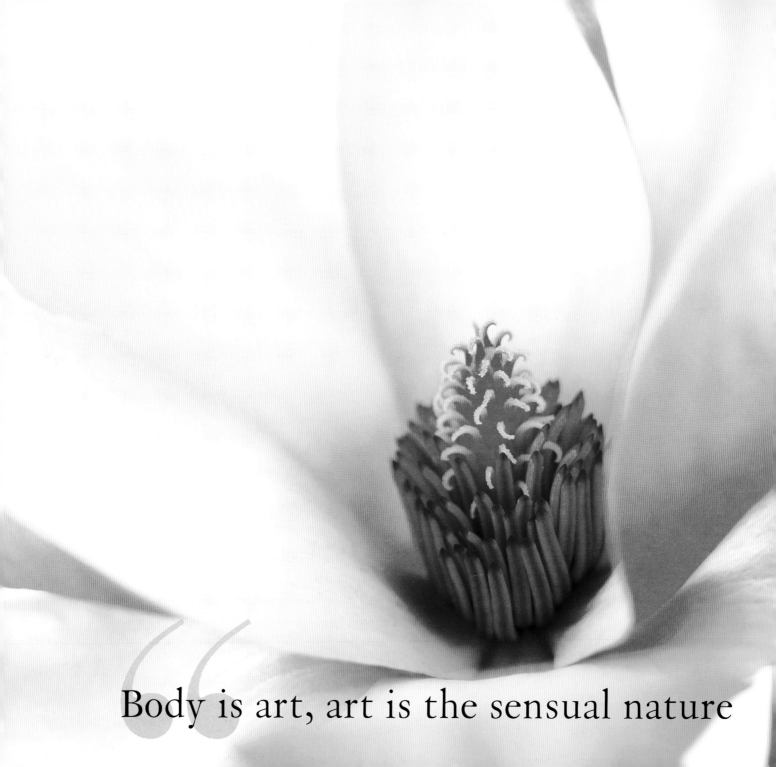

" Body is art, art is the sensual nature

organic *sexuality*

engenerated into the life of the spirit.

Bettina von Arim

Sexuality is our creative energy. Understanding the importance of sexual energy as it relates to birthing **beauty** and wellness may be the single most important thing you can do for yourself. *Terra incognita* for some, the ocean of life for others, sexuality is a subject that deserves much **exploration**. The multifaceted nature of sexuality plays an enormous role in our lives. It is one manifestation of **energy**—the libidinal type. From Tantra to soy, self-love to dang gui, fantasies to Kegels, there exists a wide variety of natural and organic approaches toward enhancing our **sexuality**. Yet our sexuality can be fraught with many misconceptions, often stemming from our upbringing and cultural influences. Our views on sexuality can be as different and **diverse** as our religious teachings, socioeconomic status, ethnic heritage, and education. ● Interestingly, if one lives life on a higher vibrational level, external constructs placed on sexual expression do not figure into the scenario. Our body is pure vibrating energy. As we access the higher vibrating levels of our being, we become more connected with **spirit**. The more connected we are with spirit, the more apt we are to ignore or at least overlook external influences in our life. ● At this more evolved point, free-flowing sexuality can fruitfully blossom, reseed itself, and continue to **flourish** throughout a lifetime.

"Sex pleasure in woman…is a kind of magic

Begin with Yourself

Reaching this higher vibrational level means that you are in a place where you have knowledge of and communication with self—or, more organically put, spirit. You should know that it all begins with the love, intimacy, and sensuality expressed first to yourself. When you know what gives you pleasure, you will more effectively communicate this special information about yourself outward.

Part of this remarkably nurturing higher plane is understanding the erotic beauty surrounding you at every given moment. Look deeply to understand how this beauty affects and arouses you. The world is astoundingly erotic. Enjoyment of the erotic is about our love for beauty. In the caves of Lascaux, there is a famous painting of the hunter who has shot an arrow into a buffalo, and the hunter has an erection. Why do you think this is? He has prayed to his God to provide food and clothing for his tribe. God has blessed him with these provisions. He has made a connection with the divine. The beautiful and mighty buffalo spirit will become one with the tribe through the food that they eat and the skins that they wear.

This is pretty heady stuff! And for this hunter, quite a turn-on. But it illustrates how we all experience varying forms of arousal as we watch life unfold. Every one of you reading this has a personal interpretation of the erotic beauty that surrounds and arouses you. What we need to learn, however, is how to recognize, respect, and connect with this form of beauty.

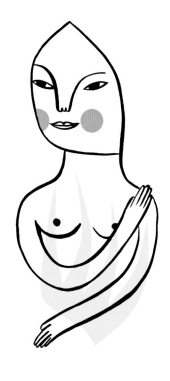

Sexuality as Universal Energy

Healing traditions from the earliest times to present include sexuality as a sacred expression of the divine. Out of the womb of creation comes our sexuality. It is the dance of life that balances, renews, regenerates, and reproduces. There is one divine, creative

spell; it demands complete abandon.

Simone de Beauvoir

energy flowing through all things, giving life. This creation is God's love flowing through and between everything.

Becoming a loving person is an integral part of living organically. This includes loving the Earth, your neighbors, your significant other, and yourself. What's more, love in the organic sense reaches beyond the traditional meaning of intimacy. It includes compassion, empathy, enchantment, sensuality, commitment, and many other emotions.

One important facet of love is our sexuality and how we express it. Blockages in our sexual energy impede our free-flowing ability to express ourselves and realize our desires. To discover and release your sexuality, you want to begin by looking inward and reflecting on who you are, why you're here, and what it is that truly makes you happy. Make clear your desires, visualize them, and give them a voice. Positively affirm your desired outcome. Fantasize to fuel the erotic imagination.

To understand your sexuality, you need to know that it begins in the mind and not the genitals. Sociocultural and religious upbringing often tarnish or repress our views of sexuality by fusing the concept on the actual act of sex. Sexuality may also be distorted through media and advertising exploitation, which send mixed messages loaded with sexual innuendoes and overtones. And of course we can't forget the fear connected to sexuality, as we associate sexuality with the act of sex and that act with potential trauma— sexually transmitted disease, unwanted pregnancy, sexual abuse, rape, and problems defining our sexual identity. Now, for good measure, let's throw in anxiety, as we struggle with our ability to have children, our ability to perform, PMS, menopause, and impotence. Clearly, the topic of sexuality can bring up many stressful issues. All the more reason to do some soul searching and open the communication channels within yourself and be-

Sexercize

In general, it's a good idea to avoid intense exercise in the evening because vigorous exercise wakes you up and can make it difficult to fall asleep. The exception is sex. The release and relaxation felt after an orgasm, when coupled with the effect of the endorphins released, produces an afterglow that is actually quite soothing and sleep-inducing.

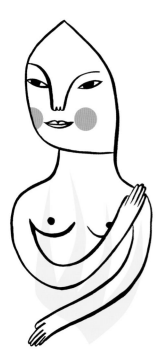

tween you and your loved ones. Only then can we see, receive, and give love in the organic sense, organically loving *all* those dear to us with compassion, empathy, enchantment, and commitment. Then we are free to add the actual act of sex and all its passion where it's appropriate to the relationship.

Sacred Sexuality

I feel that when we make love from a higher level of consciousness, we experience the sacredness, the divinity, and the exquisite pleasure of union with God. Whether it is a matter of loving yourself or your beloved, lovemaking should include a keen awareness of the sensations in your body and learning how to modulate the way in which you physically respond to these sensations. Controlling your response to these energies in your body allows for heightening of the entire experience—the merging oneness with divinity.

Whether you enjoy tantric sex or remain with your own practices, it is paramount to have regular, loving sex. The physical pleasures and benefits go without saying, and the benefits in deepening a relationship with your partner can affect your overall health and wellness. Visualize having regular, loving intimacy as an important part of your day-to-day life. If you are experiencing loss of sexual desire—and this is not a physiological problem but one of simply feeling fatigued and overextended in other areas of your life—know that you can turn this situation around. You have the will to do this. Positively affirm that you will simplify your life to be able to include regular enjoyment of your sexuality.

Enhancing Sexual Desire

If to-do lists, children, deadlines, or the hectic pace of life in general is draining your sex drive, you may want to try these healthy, gentle ways to enhance your desires and reconnect with this beautiful experience.

● Eat a whole foods, organic diet, practice stress-reduction and consciousness-raising techniques, and get plenty of physical exercise.

● Get your complex carbohydrates in fruits, veggies, and grains, and avoid sweets.

● Get enough of the following vitamins and minerals, either in your diet or through supplements: Gamma Linolenic Acid (GLA); glutathione; magnesium; vitamins A, B complex, C, E; and zinc. Your doctor can check your blood to see if any of these nutrients need to be supplemented.

● Set a mood. Indulge all the senses in the bedroom with massage oil, your favorite CDs, fresh sheets, a scented candle or aromatherapy diffuser, and fresh flowers.

● Introduce the right aromas. Research suggests a connection between sexual arousal in women and the sweet smell of Good and Plenty candy, baby powder, pumpkin pie, and lavender oil. All of these aromas caused measurable increases in vaginal blood flow, a known marker of sexual arousal. Researchers theorize that certain scents trigger mood-lightening happy memories and that these scents may also act on brain chemicals that control mood.

● If you snore a lot, seek treatment. Sleep apnea with snoring (where the airway becomes blocked during sleep and breathing briefly halts) seems to suppress proper hormone functions and diminish oxygen levels in the bloodstream. Researchers found improvements in the areas of orgasm and sexual drive after sleep apnea was successfully treated.

Self-Love

Totally organic, orgasmic, and tuned-in, masturbation or self-love can be the wellspring from which we come to know and enjoy ourselves deeply and intimately. One of the reasons that 20 percent of all women rarely experience or never have orgasm is due to never having been adequately aroused. By taking responsibility for your own arousal, you have the ability to turn this around. Self-love allows you to find out what really turns you on and makes you feel good. When you become aware in this way, you are able to enjoy a more dynamic experience, if and when you are in a relationship with someone special.

Sexual and Reproductive Health

Fulfilling your sexual needs and desires is inherently important for overall good health and thus for natural beauty. Physical, mental, and environmental stresses can potentially create great imbalances in your endocrine system—the great hormonal regulator of your body—and thus inhibit your ability to realize sexual fulfillment. Mental and chemical stresses can come from unrelenting anxiety; toxic emotions; chemicals in your food, water, and air; poor diet; and lack of exercise. Physical stress can result from perimenopause and menopause, along with poor prostate health and impotence. All of these influences can throw off the delicate hormonal balance in your body, but fortunately there are organic approaches to modulate these hormone changes. And remember, it is important to seek professional and medical support as needed.

To begin with, what a man eats can be of dramatic importance to his sexual health. For example, Danish researchers reported in 1994 in the British medical journal *The Lancet* that men who eat organic foods had twice the sperm count as those who did not eat organically.

Exposure to endocrine-disrupting chemicals (environmental estrogen) dramatically increases the incidence of testicular and prostate cancer in men, along with causing a reduced sperm count. Those same chemicals also raise the incidence of breast cancer in both women and men. (It is also interesting to note that excessive amounts of estrogen were found in premenopausal women who were heavy meat eaters, as compared to their vegetarian counterparts.)

Conversely, recent studies have found that women with high levels of phytoestrogens (plant estrogens) enjoyed a low risk for cancer. A 1992 study published in *The Lancet* confirmed that Japanese women consuming a diet rich in soy foods had concentrations of phytoestrogenic compounds that were 100 to 1,000 times higher than in American and Finnish women. All organic soy products, including tempeh and soymilk, are rich in phytoestrogens, and doctors are touting their

Sexual Therapy

Sex therapy involves behavior modification surrounding performance demands and emotions (guilt, fear, and cultural attitudes) that interfere with sexual responsiveness. It teaches new behaviors that enhance the sexual experience. Sex therapy often includes what are called sensate focus exercises. These exercises allow a couple to relate to each other physically without performance pressure or anxiety. Each partner takes a turn caressing the other, slowly progressing to genital stimulation, and if desired, genital sex. This approach allows couples to communicate nonverbally the type of stimulation they enjoy. If you seek advice from a sex therapist, make sure this person is qualified, with an advanced degree in the profession (such as a psychiatrist, psychologist, social worker, marital and family therapist, nurse, or a marriage and family counselor).

protein, antioxidant, bone-building, and cancer-preventing benefits. An important word of caution, though: Until more research can be done, women with a history of breast cancer should avoid concentrated soy protein supplements and minimize consumption of foods containing soy. The estrogen in plants, although weaker than naturally produced estrogen in the body, may spur cancer growth by creating undesirable estrogenic activity in breast tissue.

See your primary health care practitioner if you have any condition or disorder. While natural holistic approaches can often help, they are not meant to replace your doctor.

Vaginal Health

Vaginal dryness is a problem for many women. Stress, menopause, pregnancy, and nursing can all be factors. To combat vaginal dryness, try the following:

● Drink lots of water for good hydration.

● Lubricate your inner vaginal area with hormonal creams that thicken and nourish vaginal tissues. Or opt for a nonhormonal vaginal lubricant to alleviate dryness. Comfrey salves or Sylk (a natural kiwi-based lubricant) are two good options. Both are readily available in health stores.

● Apply organic olive, sesame, or sweet almond oil to moisturize your outer vaginal area.

● Make sure you're getting enough essential fatty acids in your diet; they can be very helpful in staying lubricated.

Squeeze Those Kegels

You may have been told to do Kegel exercises to help prevent urine leakage. Kegel exercises have other benefits, too. They condition and tone the vaginal muscles, increase blood circulation to this area, and ultimately help keep the tissues healthy and moist. To perform Kegels, tighten the pubococcygeus, also known as the PC muscles, that surround the vagina for 10 seconds, then relax. Repeat 10 times. Do this several times during the day. Work up to 100 or more times a day. Do them while waiting at red lights or waiting in line at the store. I do these when in yoga's "goddess" pose—lying on my back with my arms out to the side, bottoms of feet together, and knees dropped down to the sides. You might also want to try Kegels when listening to music, dancing, deep breathing, preparing a meal, or doing any beautifying ritual, such as a facial or scalp massage.

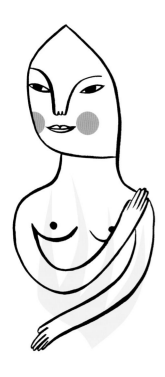

● Use organic liquid soaps to cleanse the genital area. It is simply not necessary to use harsh alkaline deodorant soaps in this area.

● Let the area breathe! Wear loose, comfortable, organic cotton or silk undergarments. Pantyhose and rayon or acrylic underthings, along with skin-tight pants, compromise the flow of life force energy through your vaginal area.

Menstruation

A woman's period represents a very powerful time of month. We are highly creative, intuitive, and introspective during this time, connecting to the creative energy of the universe. In Native American tradition, it is generally referred to as "moon time." Entrained to the lunar rhythms, this is when women are seen as intimately connected to the universal energy. We become full, just like the moon.

To optimize and fully appreciate your menstrual cycle, you may want to rethink your attitude toward menstruation. You can start by affirming and asserting positive, outflowing, creative energy during this time. Your sisters throughout history have taken this time to go inward and birth tremendous wisdom and energy. Women would go into moonhuts and be served nutritive teas and broths. Taking a cue from our sisters, try to view your menstrual cycle not as an ordeal to be gotten through, but rather as a time for self-nurturing.

Also, consider natural and organic approaches to dealing with your menstrual flow, from normal symptoms of discomfort to routine self-care.

● If you suffer menstrual cramps or experience heavy, scant, or irregular bleeding, hormonal imbalances may be the cause. Always see your primary care physician for any menstrual irregularities. In addition (and with your physician's endorsement), you can try chamomile, chasteberry, dang gui (dong quai), and gingerroot tea, all beneficial for their hormonal balancing and analgesic effects.

● Get your full complement of dietary nutrients through food choices and supplements. Optimizing your nutritional intake, when combined with efforts to get proper physical activity, reduce your stress levels, and enjoy adequate rest, will naturally act to enhance and promote menstrual regularity. And, just as a reminder, regularity implies a minimal amount of difficulties with menstruation, including tolerable cramping or generally marginal monthly discomfort.

● Cut back on saturated fats, which exacerbate cramps and put stress on the liver. Your liver helps metabolize estrogen, and excessive estrogen may cause heavy bleeding.

● You might also consider taking healthy oils. Every living cell in your body needs essential fatty acids; they are necessary for rebuilding and producing new cells. Essential fatty acids are also used by the body to product prostaglandins, hormonelike substances that act as chemical messengers and regulators for various body processes. Flaxseed and evening primrose are two of the most popular essential fatty acids.

PMS

Weeping, aggression, irritability, listlessness—they're all attributed to premenstrual syndrome, or PMS. Symptoms can also include headaches, swollen breasts, larger-than-life stress, aches, and weight gain. If you suffer mentally or physically around your moon time, consider changing your nutritional intake, physical activity, stress reduction techniques, *and* your attitude. Fluid retention is thought to be a key factor in many PMS symptoms. Daily doses of B complex, folic acid, as well as evening primrose

Aphrodisiacs

So many seductive foods beckon us. Cardamom, figs, and pomegranates are identified with the feminine, while asparagus, cucumbers, and eggplant are identified with the masculine. Truffles are said to impart a seductive power to those who eat them, while seafoods such as oysters are seen as incredible turn-ons. Other celebrated aphrodisiacs include black beans, blueberries, celery, eggs, dark mushrooms, ocean and freshwater fish, olives, and seafood. And let's not forget to include almonds, apricots, bananas, chocolate, dates, honey, licorice, and pine nuts.

Fact or fiction? Who knows. These foods, plus so many more, may enhance sexual desire and strengthen the sexual chi or energy. Eat these foods—all organic, of course—regularly, and you may strengthen your sexual vitality. At the very least, you'll have a great meal!

Understanding Menopause

Menopause actually begins with a lengthy prelude, perimenopause. This occurs for several years between a woman's mid to late 40s, and it marks the beginning of many body chemistry changes. Once menopause actually begins, physiological changes include a decline in the female hormones estrogen and progesterone and an increase in the male hormones. Most notably, levels of the male hormone testosterone increase by twentyfold with the advent of menopause. This may contribute in part to a newfound assertiveness and commitment to protecting ourselves, our loved ones, and all of life. Our ability to mother our own offspring has now transformed into a capacity to mother the world.

oil may help. Uva-ursi is also recommended to relieve bloating, as is decreased consumption of salt and caffeine. Chasteberry is a primary herbal treatment for dispelling and balancing a wide variety of menstrual problems, and dang gui may help relax the muscles of the uterus and thus decrease cramping.

Many women find aromatherapy helpful in controlling PMS. Chamomile and lavender are both quite soothing. Geranium and bergamot seem to work wonders with aggressiveness and irritability. Rose or clary sage may help during weepy, depressed times, and grapefruit is beneficial for tired or listless feelings.

Organic Menopause

Menopause is an exciting time of metamorphosis for women. It is a time to transition into and celebrate what can be the most powerful, vibrant, and fulfilling time of a women's life. As the reproductive years end, many women feel a sense of freedom that enhances sensuality and increases appreciation of sex. It's very important that women do not buy in to the notion that menopause is the end of womanhood. The wise woman sees this time as an initiation into newfound values, exceptional creativity, and social consciousness.

Having said this, it is important to understand that hormonal changes are taking place during menopause, and these changes can cause physical differences in hair and skin, energy levels, body shape and weight, and libido.

Menopause brings with it symptoms that range from mild to strong—some desirable and some not so. Not all women experience all of these symptoms, and studies indicate that a woman's attitude toward menopause can markedly increase or decrease these symptoms. Symptoms include everything from increased (or decreased) energy levels and hot flashes to sore breasts and increased (or decreased) sexual desire.

“I believe in the flesh and the body, which is

In treating symptoms of menopause, I can't emphasize enough the importance of seeing a doctor who respects your wishes, your lifestyle, and your individual situation. You want a doctor who gives you all the facts but then allows you to make any final decisions that are distinctly right for you. Together with your physician, you want to make the most informed decision possible. There are excellent books by physicians, nutritionists, and herbalists that delve into the subject of menopause, and it's a good idea to read up first so you can ask intelligent questions and communicate effectively with your doctor.

Natural Hormonal Balance

To work with the hormonal changes that occur during menopause, you want to include nourishing phytoestrogens in your diet, such as lots of organic greens (collards, dandelion, escarole, kale, mustard greens), apples, carrots, potatoes, soymilk, tofu, and yams. Increase your calcium (found in dark leafy greens, low-fat yogurt, almonds, and sesame seeds), and decrease consumption of animal foods, fried foods, dairy products, snack foods, fast foods, sugar and refined carbohydrates, caffeine, alcohol, and tobacco.

Aromatherapy may also prove beneficial in treating some menopause symptoms. Scents that seem to work particularly well include bergamot, clary sage, coriander, geranium, jasmine, and nutmeg.

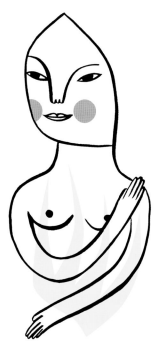

worthy of worship...
Richard Jefferies

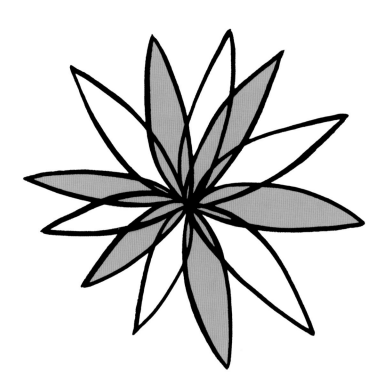

The Essence of Radiant Beauty

This, my friends, brings us to the end of the book. I hope that along the way and through these pages you discovered your own definition of beauty, whether from a spiritual, physical, emotional, or environmental perspective. Ideally, I hope your definition encompasses a bit of all four viewpoints. Most of all, it is my greatest wish that your awareness of beauty has reached new heights. Raising your level of awareness sets the stage for change, and inherent to change is letting go of old practices that may have held you back from realizing your true inner and outer beauty. As you go on from here, remember that you are empowered with the right to make choices in your life. By making organic and holistic choices, you will be able to experience and relish the essence of radiant beauty.

After all, the time and the need for organic is now. And there are certainly many ways to travel this perpetual and everlasting path in a most meaningful manner. For some of you, a slow, meditative start is best. A meditative start allows you to choose to integrate one small concept, approach, or practice from this book into your life. Others of you may choose to fully and inexorably inundate yourselves in the spirit of organic beauty and well-being. Either approach is fine. It's all part of the same thing—your evolutionary consciousness. Every one of you is on an evolutionary arc that will bring you home to the same state of being. Be as gentle, kind, and loving as you can. Know that finding challenges along this path is a sign that you are taking responsibility—for yourself, others, and the Earth. Moreover, know that by simply understanding the words I write here, you've already come a long way toward developing your own way of living an organic lifestyle.

By growing aware and living organically you become an active participant in and witness to one of the most important paradigm shifts taking place in modern times. "Think globally, act locally" never rang more true than today. Don't feel as if any of your actions are ever inconsequential, especially in view of the immense challenges that we face in our times. Any action that you take toward living organically is of great significance in the overall cumulative result of millions of others making small changes in their lives, as well. The character of our entire society is changing dramatically because of the collective and transformative ripple effect of each wave in the ocean of humanity. Our flow through the wholeness of life is founded on a unity within ourselves, with others, and with Earth. Together, let's embed ourselves in the unity and sensuousness of nature—our own and that which surrounds us. Truly, there can be no finer seduction than living an organic lifestyle and surrounding ourselves with beauty. This is the spirit of radiant beauty and wellness. Yes, you have now embarked on a spiritual quest that will permeate every facet of your life. Plunge in, immerse yourself, let yourself be seduced by the ecstasy of it all.

Using Herbs Safely

While herbs are generally safe to use and cause few, if any, side effects, researchers and specialists in natural medicine caution that you should use them responsibly. Foremost, if you are under a doctor's care for any health condition or are taking any medication, prescription or over-the-counter, don't take any herb without telling your doctor. Certain natural substances can change the way your body absorbs and processes certain medications. And if you're pregnant, don't self-treat with any natural remedy without the consent of your obstetrician or midwife. The same goes for nursing mothers and women trying to conceive.

Every product has the potential to cause adverse reactions. Below are guidelines for the herbs mentioned in this book that may be more likely than others to cause adverse reactions in some people. Though such occurrences are rare, you should be aware that they do exist, and you should immediately stop using an herb if you experience an unusual reaction. Also, don't exceed the recommended dosages—more is *not* better.

By familiarizing yourself with this list, you can enjoy the world of natural healing and use this book with confidence.

Herb	Botanical Name	Safety Guidelines and Possible Side Effects
Aloe gel	*Aloe barbadensis*	May delay wound healing; do not use gel externally on any surgical incision. Do not ingest the dried leaf gel, as it is a habit-forming laxative.
Black currant oil	*Ribes nigrum*	Generally regarded as safe.
Bloodroot	*Sanguinaria canadensis*	May cause nausea and vomiting in doses higher than 5 to 10 drops of regular-strength tincture more than twice a day. Safe when used in commercial dental products or under the guidance of a doctor or qualified herbalist.
Borage oil	*Borago officinalis*	Seed oil is generally regarded as safe.

Herb	Botanical Name	Safety Guidelines and Possible Side Effects
Burdock	*Arctium lappa*	Generally regarded as safe.
Calendula	*Calendula officinalis*	Generally regarded as safe.
Chamomile	*Matricaria recutita*	External use is generally regarded as safe. Very rarely, can cause an allergic reaction when ingested. People allergic to closely related plants such as asters, chrysanthemums, and ragweed should drink the tea with caution.
Chasteberry	*Vitex agnus-castus*	May counteract the effectiveness of birth control pills.
Comfrey	*Symphytum officinale*	For external use only. Do not use topically on deep or infected wounds because it can promote surface healing too quickly and not allow healing of underlying tissue.
Dandelion	*Taraxacum officinale*	Dandelion leaves are generally regarded as safe. If you have gallbladder disease, do not use dandelion root preparations without medical approval.
Dang gui	*Angelica sinensis*	If you suffer from a condition that may involve heavy menstrual bleeding, such as endometriosis, do not use without the guidance of a qualified practitioner.
Echinacea	*Echinacea angustifolia, E. purpurea,* and *E. pallida*	Do not use if allergic to closely related plants such as asters, chrysanthemums, and ragweed. Do not use if you have tuberculosis, or an autoimmune condition such as lupus or multiple sclerosis because echinacea stimulates the immune system.
Elderberry	*Sambucus canadensis*	Flower and ripe fruit are generally regarded as safe. Seeds, bark, leaves, and unripe fruit can cause vomiting or severe diarrhea.
	S. nigra	Flower and ripe fruit are generally regarded as safe. Unripe fruit may cause vomiting.
Evening primrose oil	*Oenothera biennis*	Generally regarded as safe.
Eyebright	*Euphrasia officinalis*	Generally regarded as safe.
Fennel seed	*Foeniculum vulgare*	Do not use medicinally for more than 6 weeks without supervision by a qualified practitioner.
Flaxseed oil	*Linum usitatissimum*	Generally regarded as safe.

(continued)

Herb	Botanical Name	Safety Guidelines and Possible Side Effects
Ginger	*Zingiber officinale*	May increase bile secretion if you have gallstones; do not use therapeutic amounts of the dried root or powder without guidance from a health-care practitioner. Generally regarded as safe when used as a spice.
Goldenseal	*Hydrastis canadensis*	Generally regarded as safe for topical use. Do not use internally if you have high blood pressure.
Green tea	*Camellia sinensis*	Generally regarded as safe. (Black tea is not recommended for excessive or long-term use because it can stimulate the nervous system.)
Hibiscus	*Hibiscus sabdariffa*	Generally regarded as safe.
Indigo, wild	*Baptisia tinctoria*	Long-term use is not recommended, except under the supervision of a qualified practitioner. Doses larger than 10 drops of tincture taken three times daily can cause vomiting and diarrhea.
Kelp	*Nereocystis luetkeana*	If you have high blood pressure or heart problems, use only once a day or less. Do not use if you have hyperthyroidism. Take with adequate liquid. Long-term use is not recommended.
Lavender	*Lavandula officinalis, L. angustifolia,* and *L. vera*	Generally regarded as safe.
Lemon	*Citrus limon*	Generally regarded as safe.
Lemongrass	*Cymbopogon citratus*	Generally regarded as safe.
Licorice	*Glycyrrhiza glabra*	Do not use if you have diabetes, high blood pressure, liver or kidney disorders, or low potassium levels. Do not use daily for more than 4 to 6 weeks because overuse can lead to water retention, high blood pressure caused by potassium loss, or impaired heart and kidney function. Deglycyrrhizinised licorice is usually free of adverse effects.
Marshmallow	*Althaea officinalis*	May slow the absorption of medications taken at the same time.

Herb	Botanical Name	Safety Guidelines and Possible Side Effects
Milk thistle	*Silybum marianum*	Generally regarded as safe.
Myrrh	*Commiphora myrrha*	Can cause diarrhea and irritation of the kidneys. Do not use if you have uterine bleeding for any reason.
Nettle	*Urtica dioica*	If you have allergies, your symptoms may worsen, so take only one dose a day for the first few days.
Parsley	*Petroselinum crispum*	Do not use if you have kidney disease, because it increases urine flow when used in therapeutic amounts. Safe as a garnish or ingredient in food.
Psyllium	*Plantago ovata*	Do not use if you have a bowel obstruction. Take 1 hour after other drugs. Take with at least 8 ounces of water.
Rhubarb (also sold as Chinese Rhubarb)	*Rheum officinale*	Do not use if you have intestinal obstruction, abdominal pain of unknown origin, or any inflammatory condition of the intestines such as appendicitis, colitis, irritable bowel syndrome, and so on. If you have a history of kidney stones, use with caution. Do not use in children less than 12 years of age. Do not use for more than 8 to 10 days.
Rosemary	*Rosmarinus officinalis*	May cause excessive menstrual bleeding in therapeutic amounts. Generally regarded as safe when used as a spice.
Sage	*Salvia officinalis*	Used in therapeutic amounts, can increase sedative side effects of drugs. Do not use if you're hypoglycemic or undergoing anticonvulsant therapy. Generally regarded as safe when used as a spice.
Stevia	*Stevia rebaudiana*	Generally regarded as safe.
Thyme	*Thymus vulgaris*	Generally regarded as safe.
Uva-ursi	*Arctostaphylos uva-ursi*	Do not use for more than 2 weeks without the supervision of a qualified practitioner. Do not use if you have kidney disease, because it contains tannins, which can cause further kidney damage. Tannins can also irritate the stomach.
Witch hazel	*Hamamelis virginiana*	Generally regarded as safe.
Yarrow	*Achillea millefolium*	Rarely, handling flowers can cause a skin rash.

Using Essential Oils Safely

Essential oils are inhaled or placed on the skin, but with few exceptions, they're never taken internally.

Most essential oils should never be applied to your skin neat (undiluted). Dilute them in a carrier base, which can be an oil (such as almond oil), cream, or gel, before application. The only exceptions are jasmine, lavender, rose, and tea tree, which you can apply undiluted.

Many essential oils may cause skin irritation or allergic reactions in people with sensitive skin. Before applying any new oil to the skin, always do a patch test. Put a few drops of the essential oil mixed with the carrier base on the back of your wrist. Wait for an hour or more. If irritation or redness occurs, wash the area with cold water. Retest using half the amount of oil. If you don't experience any irritation, just use half the amount. If you do experience irritation, avoid the oil altogether.

Here are some additional guidelines for using essential oils safely:

● Do not self-prescribe essential oils for serious medical or psychological problems.

● Do not apply essential oils to damaged or abraded skin. Damaged skin absorbs essential oils easily, making irritation, sensitization, and reactions more likely.

● Do not use essential oils during pregnancy or while nursing.

● Do not use essential oils to treat babies and infants.

● Store essential oils in dark bottles, away from light and heat, and out of reach of children and pets.

Essential Oil	Botanical Name	Safety Guidelines and Possible Side Effects
Basil	*Ocimum basilicum*	Do not use while nursing, on infants and small children, or over extended periods of time. Do not use more than three drops in the bath.
Bergamot	*Citrus bergamia*	Avoid direct sunlight while using this oil because it can cause skin sensitivity (except bergapten-free type).
Cabbage rose (also sold as pink cabbage rose)	*Rosa × centifolia*	Generally regarded as safe.
Calendula (also sold as marigold)	*Calendula officinalis*	Generally regarded as safe.
Carrot seed (also sold as Queen Anne's lace and wild carrot)	*Daucus carota*	Generally regarded as safe.
Chamomile, German	*Matricaria recutica*	Generally regarded as safe.
Chamomile, Roman	*Chamaemelum nobile*	Generally regarded as safe.
Clary sage	*Salvia sclarea*	Do not use with alcohol because it can cause lethargy and exaggerate drunkenness.
Coriander	*Coriandrum sativum*	Do not use for more than 2 weeks without the guidance of a qualified practitioner because it can cause lethargy and unconsciousness in large doses.
Damask rose (also sold as Bulgarian rose)	*Rosa × damascena*	Generally regarded as safe.
Eucalyptus (includes blue gum, broad-leaved peppermint, and lemon-scented varieties)	*Eucalyptus* var.	Do not use for more than 2 weeks without the guidance of a qualified practitioner. Do not use more than 3 drops in the bath. Do not use at the same time as homeopathic remedies. Do not apply externally to the faces of infants and young children. Can be used undiluted for dental pain.

(continued)

Essential Oil	Botanical Name	Safety Guidelines and Possible Side Effects
Frankincense	*Boswellia carteri*	Generally regarded as safe.
Geranium	*Pelargonium graveolens*	Generally regarded as safe.
Grapefruit	*Citrus × paradisi*	Generally regarded as safe.
Jasmine	*Jasminum officinale*	Generally regarded as safe.
Juniper	*Juniperus communis*	Do not use for more than 2 weeks without the guidance of a qualified practitioner because juniper is toxic at certain levels. Do not use if you have kidney disease.
Lavender	*Lavandula angustifolia*	Generally regarded as safe. Can be used undiluted, but keep it away from your eyes.
Lemon	*Citrus limon*	Do not use more than 3 drops in the bath. Avoid direct sunlight while using this oil because it can cause skin sensitivity.
Marjoram	*Origanum marjorana*	Generally regarded as safe.
Nutmeg	*Myristica fragrans*	Do not use for more than 2 weeks without the guidance of a qualified practitioner because nutmeg is toxic at certain levels. Inhale with caution; it can cause nausea.
Patchouli	*Pogostemon cablin*	Generally regarded as safe.

Essential Oil	Botanical Name	Safety Guidelines and Possible Side Effects
Peppermint	*Mentha piperita*	Do not use more than 3 drops in the bath. Do not use at the same time as homeopathic remedies. Do not get it near your eyes. Do not use it on the faces of infants and small children. Peppermint oil can be used internally, with this caution: Ingestion of peppermint essential oil may lead to stomach upset in sensitive individuals. If you have gallbladder or liver disease, do not use without medical supervision. Can be used undiluted for dental pain.
Rosemary	*Rosmarinus officinalis*	Do not use if you have hypertension. Do not use if you have epilepsy, due to this herb's powerful action on the nervous system.
Rosewood	*Aniba rosaeodora*	Generally regarded as safe. Can be used undiluted on pimples and sores.
Sandalwood	*Santalum album*	Generally regarded as safe. Can be used undiluted as a perfume, but keep it away from your eyes.
Spike lavender	*Lavandula latifolia*	Generally regarded as safe.
Tea tree	*Melaleuca alternifolia*	Generally regarded as safe. May be applied undiluted to the skin.
Ylang-ylang	*Cananga odorata* var. *genuina*	Can be used undiluted as a perfume, but keep it away from your eyes. Use in moderation because its strong smell can cause nausea or headaches.

Recommended Reading and Resources

The following information has been compiled as a starting point from which you can learn more about topics presented in this book. Listing these sources does not necessarily constitute an endorsement by Rodale Inc.

Books

Ackerman, Diane. *A Natural History of the Senses*. New York: Random House, 1990.

Alexander, Jane. *Rituals for Sacred Living*. New York: Sterling Publishing Co., Inc., 1999.

Allende, Isabel. *Aphrodite: A Memoir of the Senses*. New York: HarperFamingo, 1998.

Anand, Margo. *The Art of Sexual Magic*. New York: Putnam, 1995.

Ausubel, Kenny. *Restoring the Earth: Visionary Solutions from the Bioneers*. Tiburon, CA: H J Kramer, 1997.

Balch, James, and Phyllis A. Balch. *Prescription for Nutritional Healing*. Garden City Park, NY: Avery Pub. Group, 1998.

Berry, Thomas. *The Dream of the Earth*. San Francisco, CA: Sierra Club Books, 1988.

Borysenko, Joan. *A Woman's Book of Life: The Biology, Psychology, and Spirituality of the Feminine Life Cycle*. New York: Riverhead Books, 1996.

Breedlove, Greta. *The Herbal Home Spa: Naturally Refreshing Wraps, Rubs, Lotions, Masks, Oils, and Scrubs*. Pownal, VT: Storey Books, 1998.

Brower, Michael, and Warren Leon. *The Consumer's Guide to Effective Environmental Choices: Practical Advice from the Union of Concerned Scientists*. New York: Three Rivers Press, 1999.

Chopra, Deepak. *Ageless Body, Timeless Mind: The Quantum Alternative to Growing Old*. New York: Harmony Books, 1993.

———. *Perfect Health: The Complete Mind/Body Guide* (1st edition) New York: Three Rivers Press, 2000.

Close, Barbara. *Well Being: Rejuvenating Recipes for Body and Soul*. San Francisco, CA: Chronicle Books, 2000.

Conger, Nancy. *Sensuous Living: Expand Your Sensory Awareness*. St. Paul, MN: Llewellyn Publications, 1995.

Cruden, Loreen. *The Spirit of Place: A Workbook for Sacred Alignment*. Rochester, VT: Destiny Books, 1995.

Cunningham, Scott. *Magical Aromatherapy: The Power of Scent*. St. Paul, MN: Llewellyn Publications, 1989.

David, Marc. Nourishing Wisdom: *A Mind/Body Approach to Nutrition and Well-Being*. New York: Bell Tower, 1994.

De Luca, Diana. *Botanica Erotica: Arousing Body, Mind, and Spirit*. Rochester, VT: Healing Arts Press, 1998.

Dougans, Inge, with Suzanne Ellis. *The Art of Reflexology: A New Approach Using the Chinese Meridian Theory*. Rockport, MA: Element Books, 1992.

Douillard, John, and Martina Navratilova. *Body, Mind, and Sport: The Mind-Body Guide to Lifelong Health, Fitness, and Your Personal Best*. New York: Three Rivers Press, 2001.

Edgson, Vicki, and Ian Marber. *The Food Doctor: Healing Foods for Mind and Body*. London: Collins & Brown Ltd., 1999.

Edwards, Victoria H. *The Aromatherapy Companion*. Pownal, VT: Storey Books, 1999.

Elgin, Duane. *Voluntary Simplicity: Toward a Way of Life That Is Outwardly Simple, Inwardly Rich*. New York: Quill, 1993.

Epps, Roselyn Payne, and Susan Cobb Stewart, editors. *American Medical Women's Association Guide to Emotional Health*. New York: Dell Books, 1996.

Etcoff, Nancy. *Survival of the Prettiest: The Science of Beauty*. New York: Doubleday, 1999.

Facetti, Aldo. *Natural Beauty*. New York: Simon & Schuster, 1991.

Falconi, Dina. *Earthly Bodies and Heavenly Hair: Natural and Healthy Personal Care for Every Body*. Woodstock, NY: Ceres Press, 1998.

Fallon, Sally, with Mary G. Enig, Ph.D. *Nourishing Traditions: The Cookbook That Challenges Politically Correct Nutrition and the Diet Dictocrats* (2nd edition). Washington, DC: New Trends Publishing, Inc., 1999.

Gimbel, Theo. *The Color Therapy Workbook: The Use of Color for Health and Healing*. Boston, MA: Element Books, Inc., 1993.

Gittleman, Ann Louise, with Ann Castro. *The Living Beauty Detox Program: The Revolutionary Diet for Each and Every Season of a Woman's Life*. San Francisco, CA: Harper San Francisco, 2000.

Grossmann, Mark, and Glen Swartwout. *Natural Eye Care: An Encyclopedia*. Los Angeles: Kent Publishing, 1999.

Hampton, Aubrey. *What's in Your Cosmetics? A Complete Consumer's Guide to Natural and Synthetic Ingredients*. Tucson, AZ: Odonian Press, 1995.

Harper-Roth, Jaqulene. *Beautiful Face, Beautiful Body*. New York: Berkley Books, 2000.

Janssen, Mary Beth. *Naturally Healthy Hair: Herbal Treatments and Daily Care for Fabulous Hair*. Pownal, VT: Storey Books, 1999.

Judith, Anodea. *Wheels of Life: A User's Guide to the Chakra System*. St. Paul, MN: Llewellyn Publications, 1999.

Laux, Marcus, and Christine Conrad. *Natural Woman, Natural Menopause*. New York: HarperCollins 1997.

Lily. *Beauty, Health, and Happiness: A Way of Life.* Denver, CO: HCO Publishing, Inc., 2000.

Monte, Tom. *The Complete Guide to Natural Healing.* Collingdale, PA: Diane Publishing Co., 2000.

Moore, Thomas. *The Soul of Sex: Cultivating Life as an Act of Love.* New York: HarperCollins, 1998.

Murray, Michael, and Joseph Pizzorno. *Encyclopedia of Natural Medicine.* Rocklin, CA: Prima Publishing, 1998.

Northrup, Christiane. *Women's Bodies, Women's Wisdom: Creating Physical and Emotional Health and Healing.* New York: Bantam Books, 1998.

Raichur, Pratima, with Marian Cohn. *Absolute Beauty: Radiant Skin and Inner Harmony through the Ancient Secrets of Ayurveda.* New York: HarperCollins, 1997.

Rama, Swami, Rudolph Ballentine, and Alan Hymes. *Science of Breath: A Practical Guide.* Honesdale, PA: The Himalayan Institute Press. 1999.

Seaward, Brian Luke. *The Art of Calm: Relaxation Through the Five Senses.* Deerfield Beach, FL: Health Communications, Inc., 1999.

Siegel, Mo, and Nancy Burke. *Celestial Seasonings' Herbs for Health and Happiness: All You Need to Know.* Alexandria, VA: Time Life Books, 1999.

Sivananda Yoga Vedanta Center. *Yoga Mind & Body.* New York; London: Dorling Kindersley, 1996.

Smeh, Nikolaus J. *Health Risks in Today's Cosmetics: The Handbook for a Lifetime of Healthy Skin and Hair.* Garrisonville, VA: Alliance Publishing Company, 1994.

———. *Creating Your Own Cosmetics Naturally: The Alternative to Today's Harmful Cosmetic Products.* Garrisonville, VA: Alliance Publishing Company, 1995.

Steinman, David, and R. Michael Wisner. *Living Healthy in a Toxic World: Simple Steps to Protect You and Your Family from Everyday Chemicals, Poisons, and Pollution.* New York: Berkley Publishing, 1996.

Steinman, David, and Samuel Epstein. *The Safe Shopper's Bible: A Consumer's Guide to Nontoxic Household Products, Cosmetics and Food.* New York: Macmillan 1995.

Wall, Vicky. *The Miracle of Color Healing: Aura-Soma Therapy as the Mirror of the Soul.* London: The Aquarian Press, 1993.

Weil, Andrew. *Spontaneous Healing: How to Discover and Enhance Your Body's Natural Ability to Maintain and Heal Itself.* New York, Ballantine, 2000.

Winter, Ruth. *A Consumer's Dictionary of Cosmetic Ingredients* (5th edition). New York: Three Rivers Press, 1999.

Worwood, Valerie Ann. *The Complete Book of Essential Oils and Aromatherapy.* San Rafael, CA: New World Library, 1991.

Magazines

Natural Health
PO Box 37474
Boone, IA 50037
Phone: (800) 526-8440
Web site:
www.naturalhealth1.com

Healing Retreats and Spas
24 E. Cota Street
Santa Barbara, CA 93101
Phone: (805) 962-7107
Fax: (805) 962-1337
Web site:
www.healingretreats.com

Organic Style
33 E. Minor Street
Emmaus, PA 18098
Phone: (800) 365-3276
Web site:
www.organicstyle.com

Spa Finder
91 Fifth Avenue
New York, NY 10003
Phone: (800) 255-7727
Web site: www.spafinder.com

Spirituality and Health
PO Box 54153
Boulder, CO 80323
Phone: (800) 876-8202
Web site:
www.spiritualityhealth.com

Organic, Environmental, and Ecological Organizations and Info

Campaign to Label Genetically Engineered Foods
PO Box 55699
Seattle, WA 98155
Phone: (425) 771-4049
Fax: (603) 825-5841
Web site:
www.thecampaign.org

Consumers Union
101 Truman Avenue
Yonkers, NY 10703-1057
Phone: (914) 378-2000
Web site:
www.consumersunion.org

Environmental Working Group
1718 Connecticut Avenue NW,
Suite 600
Washington, DC 20009
Phone: (202) 667-6982
Fax: (202) 232-2592
Web site: www.ewg.org

Friends of the Earth
1025 Vermont Avenue NW
Washington, DC 20005
Phone: (877) 843-8687 or
(202) 783-7400
Fax: (202) 783-0444
Web site: www.foe.org

Greenpeace
702 H Street NW
Washington, DC 20001
Phone: (800) 326-0959
Web site: www.greenpeace.org

The Organic Alliance
400 Selby Avenue,
Suite T
St. Paul, MN 55102
Phone: (651) 265-3678
Web site: www.organic.org

Organic Consumers Association
6101 Cliff Estate Road
Little Marais, MN 55614
Phone: (218) 226-4164
Fax: (218) 226-4157
Web site: www.purefood.org

Organic Trade Association
PO Box 547
Greenfield, MA 01302
Phone: (413) 774-7511
Fax: (413) 774-6432
Web site: www.ota.com

Union of Concerned Scientists
2 Brattle Square
Cambridge, MA 02238
Phone: (617) 547-5552
Web site: www.ucsusa.org

Sources for Health, Food, Fitness, and Weight Loss

Alternative Medicine
1650 Tiburon Boulevard
Tiburon, CA 94920
Phone: (800) 515-4325
Web site:
 www.alternativemedicine.com

American Academy of Dermatology
930 N. Meacham Road
Schaumburg, IL 60173
Phone: (847) 330-0203
Web site: www.aad.org

American Association of Naturopathic Physicians
8201 Greensboro Drive,
 Suite 300
McLean, VA 22102
Phone: (703) 610-9037
Fax: (703) 610-9005
Web site: www.naturopathic.org

American Council on Exercise
5820 Oberlin Drive, Suite 102
San Diego, CA 92121-3787
Phone: (800) 825-3636
Fax: (858) 535-1778
Web site: www.acefitness.org

American Dietetic Association
216 W. Jackson Boulevard
Chicago, IL 60606-6995
Phone: (312) 899-0040
Web site: www.eatright.org

American Heart Association
7272 Greenville Avenue
Dallas, Texas 75231
Phone: (800) 242-8721
Web site:
 www.americanheart.org

American Herbalists Guild
1931 Gaddis Road
Canton, GA 30115
Phone: (770) 751-6021
Fax: (770) 751-7472
Web site: www.american
 herbalistsguild.com

American Holistic Health Association
PO Box 17400
Anaheim, CA 92817
Phone: (714) 779-6152
Web site: www.ahha.org

American Massage Therapy Association
820 Davis Street, Suite 100
Evanston, IL 60201
Phone: (847) 864-0123
Fax: (847) 864-1178
Web site: www.amtamassage.org

Colour Energy
402-55 Water Street
Vancouver, BC V6B 5K8
Canada
Phone: (604) 687-3757
Fax: (604) 687-3758
Web site: www.colourenergy.com

HealthWorld Online
171 Pier Avenue, Suite 160
Santa Monica, CA 90405
Web site: www.healthy.net

Herb Research Foundation
1007 Pearl Street, Suite 200
Boulder, CO 80302
Phone: (800) 748-2617
Fax: (303) 449-7849
Web site: www.herbs.org

Holistic Dental Association
PO Box 5007
Durango, CO 81303
Web site: www.holisticdental.org

International Institute of Reflexology
PO Box 12642
St. Petersburg, FL 33733
Phone: (727) 343-4811
Fax: (727) 381-2807
Website: www.reflexology-usa.net

National Association for Holistic Aromatherapy
2000 2nd Avenue Suite 206
Seattle, WA 98121
Phone: (888) 275-6242
Fax: (206) 770-5915
Web site: www.naha.org

National Institutes of Health
Editorial Operations Branch
9000 Rockville Pike, Building 31, Room 2B-03
Bethesda, MD 20892
Phone: (301) 496-4143
Web site: www.nih.gov

National Mental Health Association
1021 Prince Street
Alexandria, VA 22314-2971
Phone: (703) 684-7722
Fax: (703) 684-5968
Web site: www.nmha.org

National Sanitation Foundation International Consumer Drinking Water Information
PO Box 130140
Ann Arbor, MI 48113-0140
Telephone: (734) 769-8010
Fax: (734) 769-0109
Web site: www.nsf.org

OneBody
2000 Powell Street, #555
Emeryville, CA 94608
Phone: (888) 646-5729
Web site: www.onebody.com

Portable Practitioner
PO Box 2095
Petoskey, MI 49770
Phone: (231) 347-8591
Web site: www.portable practitioner.com

Society for Women's Health Research
1828 L Street, NW, Suite 625
Washington, DC 20036
Phone: (202) 223-8224
Fax: (202) 833-3472
Web site: www.womens-health.org

The Chopra Center for Well Being
7630 Fay Avenue
La Jalla, CA 92037
Phone: (858) 551-7788
Fax: (858) 551-7811
Web site: www.chopra.com

U.S. Department of Health and Human Services
200 Independence Avenue SW
Washington, DC 20201
Phone: (877) 696-6775
Web site: www.healthfinder.gov

United States National Library of Medicine
8600 Rockville Pike
Bethesda, MD 20894
Phone: (301) 496-4000
Web site: www.nlm.nih.gov

Sources for Organic, Holistic Beauty and Healthy Living Products

Aubrey Organics
4419 North Manhattan Avenue
Tampa, FL 33614
Phone: (800) 282-7394
Fax: (813) 876-8166
Web site: www.aubrey-organics.com

Aveda
4000 Pheasant Ridge Drive
Blaine, MN 55449
Phone: (800) 328-0849
Web site: www.aveda.com

Better Botanicals
335 Victory Drive
Herndon, VA 20170
Phone: (703) 481-3300
Fax: (703) 481-7459
Web site: www.betterbotanicals.com

Devita Natural Skin Care Systems
6845 W. Mcknight Loop, Suite A
Glendale, AZ 85308
Phone: (602) 978-8224
Web site: www.devita.net

Indian Meadow Herbals
RR1, Box 547
Eastbrook, ME 04634
Phone: (207) 565-3010
Fax: (207) 565-3402
Web site: www.imherbal.com

Jurlique
2714 Apple Valley Road
Atlanta, GA 30319
Phone: (800) 854-1110
Web site: www.jurlique.com

Lily of Colorado
PO Box 12471
Denver, CO 80212
Phone: (800) 333-5459
Web site:
    www.lilyofcolorado.com

Lush Fresh Handmade Cosmetics
8739 Heather Street
Vancouver, BC V6P 3T1
Canada
Phone: (888) 733-5874
Web site: www.lushcanada.com

Modern Organic Products (MOP)
1732 Champa Street
Denver, CO 80202
Phone: (800) 598-2739
Fax: (303) 292-9851
www.americancrew.com

Oshadi USA
1340-G Industrial Avenue
Petaluma, CA 94952
Phone: (888) 674-2344
Web site: www.oshadhiusa.com

Sundãri
379 West Broadway
New York, NY 10012
Phone: (800) 552-0203
Web site: www.sundari.com

Trillium Herbal Company
185 E. Walnut Street
Sturgeon Bay, WI 54235
Phone: (920) 746-5207
Fax: (920) 746-7649
Web site: www.bodypolish.com

Uncle Harry's Natural Products
704 228th Avenue NE
Redmond, WA 98053
Phone: (425) 643-4664
Fax: (425) 895-9391
Web site: www.uncleharrys.com

Vermont Soapworks
616 Exchange Street
Middlebury, VT 05753
Phone: (802) 388-4302
Fax: (802) 388-7471
Web site:
    www.vermontsoap.com

Weleda
175 North Route 9W
Congers, NY 10920
Phone: (800) 241-1030
Web site: www.weleda.com

Zia Natural Skin Care
1337 Evans Avenue
San Francisco, CA 94124
Phone: (800) 334-7546
Web site: www.zianatural.com

Organic Feminine and Personal Care Products and Info

Keepers! Inc.
PO Box 12648
Portland, OR 97212
Phone: (800) 799-4523
Fax: (503) 284-9883
Web site: www.gladrags.com

Lunapads International
Suite 504-825 Granville
    Street
Vancouver, BCV6Z 1K9
Canada
Phone: (604) 681-9953
Fax: (604) 681-9904
Web site: www.lunapads.com

Organic Essentials
822 Baldridge Street
O'Donnell, TX 79351
Phone: (806) 428-3486
Fax: (806) 428-3486
Web site:
    www.organicessentials.com

Holistic and Organic Companies

Alternatives for Simple Living
PO Box 2787
Sioux City, IA 51106
Phone: (800) 821-6123
Fax: (712) 274-1402
Web site:
    www.simpleliving.org

As We Change
6255 Ferris Square, Suite F
San Diego, CA 92121-3232
Phone: (858) 456-8333
Fax: (858) 456-8340
Web site:
    www.aswechange.com

Gaiam
360 Interlocken Boulevard,
Suite 300
Broomfield, CO 80021
Phone: (303) 464-3600
Fax: (303) 464-3700
Web site: www.gaiam.com

Gold Mine Natural Foods Company
7805 Arjons Drive
San Diego, CA 92126
Phone: (800) 475-3663
Web site: www.goldmine
    naturalfood.com

Harvest Direct
PO Box 50906
Knoxville, TN 37950
Phone: (865) 539-6305
Fax: (865) 539-2737
Web site: www.harvestdirect.com

Healthy Trader
647 Camino de Los Mares
    #108 PMB#191
San Clemente, CA 92673
Phone: (800) 636-2584
Fax: (949) 369-0726
Web site: www.healthytrader.com

Isabella
2780 Via Orange Way, Suite B
Spring Valley, CA 91978
Phone: (888) 481-6745
Fax: (619) 670-5203
Web site:
    www.Isabellacatalog.com

Lifekind Products
PO Box 1774
Grass Valley, CA 95945
Phone: (800) 284 4983
Web site: www.lifekind.com

Mountain Ark Trading Company
799 Old Leicester Highway
Asheville, NC 28806
Phone: (800) 643-8909
Web site:
    www.mountainark.com

Yoga Site
154 Walker Road
West Orange, NJ 07052
Phone: (877) 964-2748
Web site: yogasite.com

Index

psychological influence of, 58–59

relaxing, 71–72

rinses for, 63–64

scalp health and, 62–63

symbolism of, 58

waving, 71–72

Hair-care products

adding organic ingredients to, 66–67, 70, 102

antiseptics in, 66

for chemically treated hair, 72

conditioner, 65–66

hair spray, 72

homemade rinses, 63–64

natural preservatives in, 66

shampoo, 65–66

Hair loss

aromatherapy for, 66

causes of, 60

Hair rinses, homemade, 63–64

Hair sprays, 72

Hands

care of, 84–85

causes of discomfort of, 82–83

outdoor protection for, 85

stretching exercises for, 83–84

Hangnails, 87

Health, beauty and, 8–9

Hearing, 104–6

Herbs, safety guidelines for and possible side effects of, *126–29. See also specific herbs*

Hibiscus, as hair color rinse, 73

Holistic products, 5–6

Honey

in facial mask, 51

for hand care, 85

Hormonal creams, for vaginal lubrication, 119

Hormonal imbalances, 118, 120

Hormone replacement therapies, for aging skin, 40

Humectants, moisturizing with, 48, 49

Hydrogen peroxide, for earwax buildup, 105

I

Indigo, as hair color rinse, 73

Ingrown toenails, 88

Iron

for eyesight, 97

for lips, 107

sources of, 42

J

Jasmine oil, for menopause, 123

Jojoba oil

for cuticles, 89

for eye massage, 99

Juniper oil

for foot perspiration, 81

for stuffy nose, 99–100

K

Kegel exercises, 119

L

Lavender

for foot care, 80

in hair rinse, 64

for nail care, 87

oil

for carpal tunnel syndrome, 84

for foot perspiration, 81

for nail and cuticle care, 87

for PMS, 122

properties of, 103

as skin toner, 48

Lemon, as skin toner, 48

Lemongrass, in hair rinse, 64

Lip balms, 107

Lips, protecting, 106–7

Lipstick, harmful ingredients in, 107

Love, in organic living, 115, 116

M

Magnesium

for dental care, 109

for enhancing sexual desire, 117

sources of, 42

Manicures, 87–88

Marjoram oil, for carpal tunnel syndrome, 84

Masks, facial, 35, 39

homemade, 51, 52

Massage

aromatherapy, 101

benefits of, 52–53

for carpal tunnel syndrome, 84

eye, 96, 99

foot, 76, 79

gum, 109

hand, 76, 85

oil for, 53

self-, technique for, 53–55

Masturbation, 117

Mature skin, 40, 49

Meditation, 26–27, 95

Menopause, 122–23

skin changes in, 40

Menstruation, 120–21

Milk

as eye treatment, 97

Milk (continued)
    in facial mask, 51
    as hand soak, 85
Milk thistle, for eyesight, 96
Mindfulness, 9, 24
Moisturizing
    feet, 77
    hands, 77, 84–85
    nails, 86–87
    in skin-care regimen, 35,
        48–49
Morning ritual, 22
Mouth, 106
Mouthwash, homemade, 108
Music, effects of, 104–5

N
Nail polish, choosing, 88
Nails
    care of, 86–89
    indicating health conditions,
        86
    nutrients for, 42
Nakedness, 38
Nettles
    for hair care, 64, 70
    as skin toner, 48
Normal hair, conditioner for, 68
Normal skin, care of, 37
Nose
    function of, 99
    stuffy, 99–100
Nudity, 38
Nutmeg oil, for menopause, 123
Nutrients, for healthy skin, hair,
    and nails, 42
Nutrition
    for eyes, 97
    for hair and scalp, 61–62
    for menstrual regularity, 121

for nails, 86
for sexual health, 117,
    118–19
for skin, 41–43
for teeth, 108–9
in menopause, 123

O
Oatmeal, in facial mask, 51
Oily hair
    conditioner for, 68
    rinse for, 64
Oily skin
    care of, 38–39
    cleansers for, 47
    facial mask for, 51
    massage oils for, 53
Olive oil
    for dandruff, 63
    for eye massage, 99
    for gum massage, 109
    for lashes and brows, 99
    in salt scrub, 52
    for vaginal moisture, 119
Omega-3 fatty acids, for healthy
    hair, 61
Organic, definitions of, 14–15
Organic beauty, 2, 4, 5,
    20–21
Organic farming, 16–17
Organic foods, certified, 17
Organic lifestyle
    consciousness in, 15–16
    leading to beauty, 12–13, 15

P
Papaya, in facial mask, 51
Patch test, for identifying
    allergic reactions, 48
Pedicures, 87–88

Peppermint
    for foot care, 80
    oil, uses for, 104
Perspiration, foot, controlling,
    80–81
Pesticide use, statistics on, 15
Phytoestrogens
    for cancer prevention,
        118–19
    for menopause, 123
Pineapple, in facial mask, 51
PMS, 121–22
Positive affirmations, affecting
    health, 9
Potato slices, as eye treatment,
    97
Premenstrual syndrome (PMS),
    121–22
Protein
    for eyesight protection, 97
    sources of, 42

Q
Quercetin, for eye allergies, 98

R
Reading, recommended,
    134–37
Resources, 137–41
Rhythms of nature, 16, 94
Rosebuds, for nail care, 87
Rosemary
    in hair rinse, 64, 73
    oil
        for foot perspiration, 81
        uses for, 104
Rose oil
    for nail care, 87
    for PMS, 122
    uses for, 104